PERGAMON INTERNAT
of Science, Technology, Enginee
The 1000-volume original paperback li
industrial training and the enjc
Publisher: Robert Maxw

BIOMEDICAL ASPECTS OF LACTATION

Publisher's Notice to Educators

THE PERGAMON TEXTBOOK INSPECTION COPY SERVICE

An inspection copy of any book published in the Pergamon International Library will gladly be sent without obligation for consideration for course adoption or recommendation. Copies may be retained for a period of 60 days from receipt and returned if not suitable. When a particular title is adopted or recommended for adoption for class use and the recommendation results in a sale of 12 or more copies, the inspection copy may be retained with our compliments. If after examination the lecturer decides that the book is not suitable for adoption but would like to retain it for his personal library, then our Educators' Discount of 10% is allowed on the invoiced price. The Publishers will be pleased to receive suggestions for revised editions and new titles to be published in this important International Library.

Other titles of Interest

BAKER & REUTER:
Calcium Movement in Excitable Cells

WHITE & THORSON
The Kinetics of Muscle Contraction

INGLIS:
A Textbook of Human Biology, 2nd Edition

BUCKETT:
Introduction to Animal Husbandry

DILLON:
The Analysis of Response in Crop and Livestock Production

DODSWORTH:
Beef Production

LAWRIE
Meat Science, 2nd Edition

NELSON:
An Introduction to Feeding Farm Livestock

PARKER:
Health & Disease in Farm Animals, 2nd Edition

PRESTON & WILLIS:
Intensive Beef Production, 2nd Edition

ROSE:
Agricultural Physics

YEATES *et al.*:
Animal Science: Reproduction, Climate, Meat and Wool

The terms of our inspection copy service apply to all the above books. Full details of all books listed and specimen copies of journals listed will gladly be sent upon request.

PERGAMON STUDIES IN THE LIFE SCIENCES

BIOMEDICAL ASPECTS OF LACTATION

WITH SPECIAL REFERENCE TO LIPID METABOLISM AND MEMBRANE FUNCTIONS OF THE MAMMARY GLAND

S. PATTON

and

R. G. JENSEN

PERGAMON PRESS
OXFORD · NEW YORK · TORONTO
SYDNEY · PARIS · FRANKFURT

U.K.	Pergamon Press Ltd., Headington Hill Hall, Oxford OX3 0BW, England
U.S.A.	Pergamon Press Inc., Maxwell House, Fairview Park, Elmsford, New York 10523, U.S.A.
CANADA	Pergamon of Canada Ltd., P.O. Box 9600, Don Mills M3C 2T9, Ontario, Canada
AUSTRALIA	Pergamon Press (Aust.) Pty. Ltd., 19a Boundary Street, Rushcutters Bay, N.S.W. 2011, Australia
FRANCE	Pergamon Press SARL, 24 rue des Ecoles, 75240 Paris, Cedex 05, France
WEST GERMANY	Pergamon Press GmbH, 6242 Kronberg-Taunus, Pferdstrasse 1, Frankfurt-am-Main, West Germany

Copyright © Pergamon Press 1976

All Rights Reserved. No part of this publication may be reproduced, stored in a retrieval system or transmitted in any form or by any means: electronic, electrostatic, magnetic tape, mechanical, photocopying, recording or otherwise, without permission in writing from the publishers

Originally published in *Progress in the Chemistry of Fats and other Lipids* (Ed. R. T. Holman) Volume 14 Part 4. Reprinted here with slight revision and additions.

First edition 1976

Library of Congress Cataloging in Publication Data

Patton, Stuart.
  Biomedical aspects of lactation.

(Pergamon studies in the life sciences)
Revision of Lipid metabolism and membrane functions of the mammary gland originally published in Progress in the chemistry of fats and other lipids, v. 14, pt. 4.
Bibliography: p.
  1. Lactation. 2. Lipid metabolism. 3. Mammary glands. I. Jensen, Robert Gordon, 1926– joint author. II. Title. [DNLM: 1. Lactation. 2. Mammae-Physiology. 3. Lipids-Metabolism. 4. Breast-Physiology. WO825 P322b]
QP246.P35   1976   612.6'64   75-42461
ISBN 0-08-020192-X

Printed in Great Britain by A. Wheaton & Co., Exeter

BIOMEDICAL ASPECTS OF LACTATION

WITH SPECIAL REFERENCE TO LIPID METABOLISM AND MEMBRANE FUNCTIONS OF THE MAMMARY GLAND

CONTENTS*

PREFACE	viii
I. INTRODUCTION	1
A. Importance of the mammary gland	1
1. Biomedical considerations	2
2. Industrial considerations	2
3. Sex	3
B. The nature of milk	3
1. Species variations	3
2. Milk components	4
(a) Milk lipids	5
(b) Casein	6
(c) Whey proteins	6
(d) Other components	7
C. General relationship of lipids to lactation	7
II. RELATIONSHIP OF GENERAL BODY METABOLISM TO THAT OF THE MAMMARY GLAND	8
A. General metabolism	8
B. The rumen	11
1. Volatile fatty acids	12
2. Microbial lipids	12
3. Biohydrogenation	13
4. Polyunsaturation of milk fat	14
5. Unusual fatty acids	15
C. The serum lipoproteins	16
1. Composition and metabolism	16
2. Contribution to milk lipids	19
D. Depressed milk fat	21

*Sections I–IV were prepared by Stuart Patton and Section V was prepared by Robert G. Jensen.

III. STRUCTURE AND FUNCTION OF MAMMARY EPITHELIUM ... 22
   A. General features of the mammary gland ... 22
      1. Adipose tissue ... 23
   B. The alveolus ... 24
   C. Differentiation of the mammary epithelial cell ... 25
   D. Mammary lipid metabolism in relation to breast cancer ... 27
   E. Lactation and the functioning of cell membranes ... 29
      1. Vectoring of biosynthetic products within the cell ... 30
      2. Membrane transformation and flow within the cell ... 31
      3. Membrane aging ... 31
      4. Synthesis of the major milk constituents ... 34
         (a) The milk proteins ... 35
         (b) Lactose ... 36
         (c) Fat ... 36
      5. Milk secretion ... 39
         (a) Golgi vesicle mechanism ... 40
         (b) Milk fat globule secretion mechanism ... 42
      6. Membrane material in skim milk ... 42
      7. Composition of membranes from lactating tissue ... 43
         (a) Membrane preparation ... 43
         (b) Lipid composition of membranes ... 44
         (c) Protein composition of membranes ... 46
   F. Critique of observations of secretory phenomena ... 46
      1. Golgi secretory process ... 46
      2. Fat globule secretion ... 47
      3. Fat globule membrane ... 48
      4. Globule crescents ... 50
      5. Sidedness of plasma membrane ... 50

IV. BIOCHEMICAL PATHWAYS IN TISSUE AND MILK LIPID SYNTHESIS ... 51
   A. Introduction ... 51
   B. Energy metabolism of mammary tissue ... 52
   C. Fatty acid synthesis ... 53
      1. Enzymes ... 54
      2. Sources of carbon and pathways ... 55
      3. δ-hydroxy- and β-keto-fatty acids ... 57
      4. Pattern of milk fatty acids ... 57
   D. Triglyceride synthesis ... 58
      1. Glycerol-3-phosphate pathway ... 59
      2. Monoglyceride pathway ... 60
      3. Other pathways ... 62
      4. Properties of the triglycerides ... 62
   E. Synthesis of phospholipids and glycolipids ... 63
      1. Phospholipids ... 64
      2. Glycolipids ... 66
   F. Cholesterol ... 66

	1. Functions and metabolism of cholesterol	67
	2. Occurrence of cholesterol in milk	70
	3. Origins of milk cholesterol	72
G.	Vitamin A	74
H.	Lipogenesis in milk and milk as a living system	75
I.	Biosynthesis of milk lipids in relation to milk technology and food value	76

V. COMPOSITION OF MILK LIPIDS 77
   A. Lipid classes 78
      1. Composition 78
      2. Triacylglycerols 78
         (a) Methods of analysis 79
         (b) Structure 82
      3. Other acylglycerols 83
      4. Phospholipids 84
      5. Sterols 85
      6. Hydrocarbons 86
      7. Lipoproteins 86
   B. Composition of lipid classes 87
      1. Determination of fatty acids 87
      2. Fatty acids in general 88
      3. Protected milk 93
      4. Phospholipids 95
      5. Sphingolipids 99
      6. Sterol esters 102
   C. Summary 102

ACKNOWLEDGEMENTS 103

REFERENCES 103

ADDENDUM 111

PREFACE

Research interest in the mammary gland has grown steadily during the past two decades. While concern regarding breast cancer has been partly responsible, there are other important factors. Life and health are dependent on food, and milk, the product of the mammary gland, is one of the best. In addition the mammary gland is proving to be a very fruitful site for study of cell differentiation, metabolism and membrane phenomena. As an exterior appendage the mammary gland is easily accessible compared to many other tissues; the fact that milk provides a record of cell and tissue metabolism also is advantageous; and the normal and continuous secretion of enzymes, membranes and various cell types into milk provides a most unique opportunity for furthering the understanding of these several levels of life. For example, the milk fat globule is secreted from the lactating cell by envelopment in plasma membrane, the limiting membrane of cells. The plasma membrane is increasingly recognized as an "intelligence" of the cell, one that plays a vital role in transport, secretion, differentiation, replication and immune properties. Milk fat globules are assisting in the answer to such questions as: where do membranes come from, how are they changed from one into another, and what are their structures and functions?

This monograph is meant to be a teaching aid. It represents an effort to concentrate and unify contemporary information on the lactating mammary gland. It provides a useful entrée to the literature (including an Addendum, over 400 references). It is hoped that the level of treatment will suit senior undergraduate and beginning graduate courses serving biologists, physiologists, medical and premedical students as well as animal and dairy science students. It has purposely been kept modest in size since there are a number of extensive advanced treaties on the subject.

We are indebted to Professor R. T. Holman, who edited the original version, originally published under the title "Lipid Metabolism and Membrane Functions of the Mammary Gland", in *Progress in the Chemistry of Fats and Other Lipids*, Vol. 14, Part 4. In preparing the present version this material has been updated both in the text and in relevant recent literature.

July 1975   STUART PATTON

BIOMEDICAL ASPECTS OF LACTATION

WITH SPECIAL REFERENCE TO LIPID METABOLISM AND MEMBRANE FUNCTIONS OF THE MAMMARY GLAND

STUART PATTON

Division of Food Science and Industry,
The Pennsylvania State University,
University Park, Pennsylvania 16802

and

ROBERT G. JENSEN

Department of Nutritional Sciences,
The University of Connecticut,
Storrs, Connecticut 06268

I. INTRODUCTION

A. Importance of the mammary gland: a locus of food, sex and cancer

The mammary gland is an arrangement of the circulatory system and specialized tissues enabling the synthesis and secretion of milk, the product for nourishment of all young mammals including the human infant. Virtually all of the latter are nursed naturally or on a bottled formula based on cow's milk. Even in the relatively rare cases of milk allergy in the young human it is necessary to emulate milk in constructing a satisfactory diet formula.

It is well known, of course, that a huge industry is predicated on the product of the bovine mammary gland and that this industry makes a strong contribution to man's health and well being. Because milk is fundamentally important in our culture, lactation has been the subject of a tremendous research effort, especially at agricultural institutions throughout the world. However, it is an anachronism that this effort until very recent years was limited to investigations of milk and factors in the management of the animal that influence the quantity and quality of milk produced. The crucial machinery in all this, the mammary gland, while not totally ignored, has had to wait for the rise in science of biochemistry and physiology. That day has truly come and the marvels of lactation at the cellular and molecular levels are being revealed increasingly. This vigorous expansion of knowledge forms the basis of this monograph.

1. Biomedical considerations

It would appear that integration of knowledge in this area is timely for several reasons. It is important for biomedical purposes to be able to compare how the various tissues in the body function. As a tissue, mammary epithelium is quite remarkable in that it yields a readily accessible product, milk, which is a record of the cell's metabolism. Not only do the products of synthesis emerge from the lactating cell but also some of the cells and their machinery (enzymes and membranes) as well. From the standpoint of lipid metabolism, this is like an adipose tissue cell except with a "back door" for getting rid (secretion) of product. In fact the mammary gland is a very useful model for the study of transport phenomena. In general, molecules of many sizes, shapes and properties are transported and transformed across at least four membranes in moving from blood to milk.

Another important reason for drawing mammary metabolic information together concerns the problem of breast cancer. Lactation is a normal differentiation of mammary epithelium, while mammary cancer is not. The hormone prolactin appears to be an important stimulus in both processes.[37,179] Further, there are suggestive relationships between mammary cancer and milk-born viruses.[360] So in attacking this complex and serious problem of the human it should be of value to describe the condition of the mammary tissue in full healthy function as well as in its pathology.

A further interesting biomedical aspect of the mammary gland concerns aging. It appears that the development of mammary epithelial cells for lactation is a terminal process. Once the cell achieves the differentiated state of lactation it will never perform any other function. After a certain point early in lactation, there is little further DNA (cell) production.[11,77,355] Virtually all the cells that will produce milk for the lactation are there. Interestingly, in the human and some other species (notably ruminants) lactation can be protracted for as much as four or five years, although the yields of milk by the end of such times are very small indeed. The essential is that milk continue to be removed regularly from the gland. These lactating cells appear to be antique and they, as well as their secretion, represent an opportunity to study aging phenomena at the cellular level.

2. Industrial considerations

The added knowledge of milk which is resulting from increased research on its synthesis is assisting the dairy industry. Many of the practical problems in the processing of milk and milk products have arisen from a lack of knowledge about milk itself, particularly as a product of cell metabolism. For example, a tremendous research and development effort was lavished on dry whole milk during and following World War II in an effort to produce a beverage for the military that would be essentially indistinguishable from the fresh fluid milk. Despite the manipulation of every conceivable processing and storage variable, the product could not be improved beyond a certain point which by hindsight involved unknown properties of the milk itself, more particularly, for example, the spontaneous rearrangement of hydroxy-fatty acids to lactones that contributed off flavor. The biochemistry of this problem is discussed subsequently (p. 57); for a review, see Dimick *et al.*[85] This example is one of a number from the field of dairy research which illustrates the practical merits of basic research. In the instance cited, no doubt time, effort and money were wasted for want of some

INTRODUCTION

basic information on milk, and even though such research was mounted belatedly it has been better late than never in aiding improvement of flavor of dairy products, and related foods.

3. *Sex*

While the sexual implications of mammary gland structure and function are beyond the scope of this treatise, in emphasizing the pervasive importance of the gland it seems appropriate to note such ramifications. Non-lactating human breasts contain significant and variable amounts of adipose tissue which influences their size and shape. One probable result of the tremendous amount of research on lipid metabolism will be an understanding of what regulates lipid storage in the various tissues of the body. If this can be regulated tissue by tissue it is obvious that measures will be at hand for more precisely controlling the size and shape of the human breast. There is increasing evidence that the hormone, prolactin, regulates serum lipid uptake by the lactating mammary gland (see Addendum).

Lactation and nursing the infant involve a woman in experiences and sensations that can be fundamental in the quality of her life (Fig. 1).

B. *The nature of milk*

The function of the mammary epithelial cell is to make and secrete milk. It is the cell membranes that synthesize, assemble and secrete the components. These membranes are primarily composed of lipids and proteins. Since some of the cell membranes and proteins pass into milk as a result of the secretory processes, it is necessary to consider the synthesis and secretion of milk in order to understand metabolism of the tissue. While there is extensive information on the composition, biochemistry and ultrastructure of milk, [154,198,209,306,369] it will suffice here to discuss general attributes of milk components so that the entities being synthesized and secreted by the cell will be understood.

1. *Species variations*

Most of what is known about milk derives from studies of cow's (*Bos taurus*) milk and any dissertation on milk or the mammary gland would have to rely heavily on the knowledge of the bovine species. To a lesser yet important extent, the goat, rat, mouse and guinea pig have been employed in lactation research. For various reasons the human has not been studied extensively with respect to the biochemistry and physiology of lactation, and, of course, it is the species of utmost importance. With the surge in research on breast cancer we can expect some of the deficit in knowledge of the human mammary gland to be made up.

Presumably the information we have from the foregoing species and across species lines allows us to make some generalizations about the synthesis and secretion of milk. But it must be remembered that in this monograph we are usually writing in terms of the domestic cow and a few other experimental species. Data on milk composition for a number of species have been compiled by Jenness and Sloan.[155] In the interest of demonstrating some similarities and differences in the gross composition of milks, data for several species given in their review are presented in Table 1. The principal differences, which are relatively small, between cow's milk and human milk concern levels of protein, particularly casein, which is lower in human milk, and contents of lactose which is higher in human milk than in cow's milk. Note also the profound

TABLE 1. *Composition of Milks from Selected Mammals*[a]

	Fat	Casein	Whey protein	Lactose	Ash	Water
			%			
Human	3.8	0.4	0.6	7.0	0.2	87.6
Cow	3.7	2.8	0.6	4.8	0.7	87.3
Goat	4.5	2.5	0.4	4.1	0.8	86.8
Rat (Norway)	10.3	6.4	2.0	2.6	1.3	79.0
Guinea pig	3.9	6.6	1.5	3.0	0.8	83.6
Fur seal	53.3	4.6	4.3	0.1	0.5	34.6
Sea lion	36.5	13.8		0.0	0.0	47.3

[a] Data from ref. 155.

difference shown in the table between the composition of milks of the fur seal and sea lion and that of the other species. The virtual absence of lactose, apparently due to little or no α-lactalbumin, the B protein of lactose synthetase in the mammary tissue of these two mammals, appears to be characteristic of the pinnepeds in general as does high fat, protein and total solids (low water) in their milks. The reasons for this composition may involve the young pinneped's need for insulation, storable energy and metabolic water, all of which may be supplied more effectively by fat than by lactose. Moreover, adult pinnepeds are adapted to fish as a diet and it supplies little carbohydrate, so there would seem to be little purpose in adjusting the young animal to an exogenous supply of carbohydrate. In addition, the young seal is essentially abandoned by his mother, and for a period of time while he learns to swim and fish he must literally live off the fat of his back which came from milk and more precisely from fish (oil) which his mother converted to part of her milk fat. The author (S.P.) has had the privilege of observing baby elephant seals on the beach at Guadalupe Island (Mexico). These youngsters resemble overgrown rugby balls and they have been "blown up" by milk fat from their mother's mammary glands. This raises the consideration of diet as an important species-related factor in milk lipid composition. The subject is discussed in a subsequent section on the general metabolism of the lactating animal.

2. *Milk components*

Milk is a watery fluid and the principal component of nearly all milks is water. The material not in solution and capable of reflecting light is comprised of fat globules and casein micelles. The latter are phosphoprotein aggregates. The balance of the milk proteins are known as the whey proteins because they are left in the whey when the curd (casein) is removed by rennet (enzyme) coagulation. Other principal components contained in solution are lactose (4-O-β-galacto-pyranosyl-glucose), the milk salts and a complex mixture of organic compounds, including water-soluble vitamins, at trace levels. In some milks, tricalcium phosphate is present in suspension and associated with the casein micelles. A variety of carbohydrates occur in the milks of the various mammals, usually at levels far below that of lactose. Much of this carbohydrate is contained in glycoproteins and glycolipids.

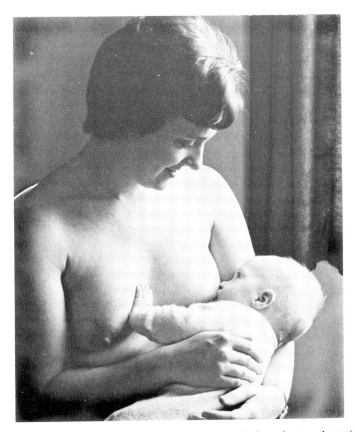

FIG. 1. Development and functioning of the mammary system is dependent on the action of diverse hormones: estrogen and progesterone from the ovaries and placenta, insulin from the pancreas, hydrocortisone from the adrenals, prolactin from the pituitary. (Photo courtesy of Robert S. Beese, the Pennsylvania State University).

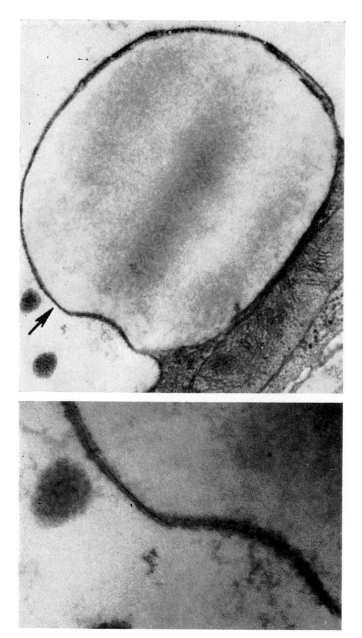

Fig. 3. Milk fat globule (rat) in process of being secreted from cell. Large mitochondrion lies under globule inside cell. Two casein micelles are evident in alveolar lumen (upper left by arrow). Note variable thickness of globule membrane. At one point (arrow) well-resolved unit membrane flush against core is evident. Globule is $1.60 \times 1.27\ \mu$ in long and short diameters. Lower figure magnifies membrane in vicinity of arrow. (Electron micrograph courtesy of P. S. Stewart.)

INTRODUCTION

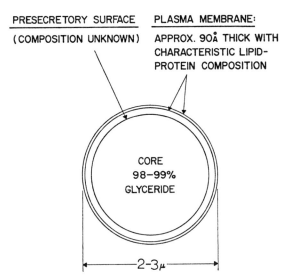

FIG. 2. Scheme for a typical milk fat globule (Patton[269]).

A comprehensive treatise[240] on the milk proteins, their chemistry and molecular biology is available. Our need here is to describe these proteins sufficiently to provide a basis for understanding the synthesis and secretion of milk in relation to metabolism of the mammary gland.

With the discovery by Brodbeck and Ebner[52] that one of the whey proteins, α-lactalbumin, is part of the lactose synthetase enzyme,* functions in milk synthesis have been sought for other milk constituents, notably β-lactoglobulin. Thus far none has been found. Casein obviously is of nutritional importance to the new-born by virtue of its curd-forming properties, as well as its calcium, phosphorus, and essential amino acid contents. The lipase activity associated with casein micelles may also have some value in nutrition of the young. Since β-lactoglobulin appears to occur only in ruminant milks, the possibility that it has an exclusive role in the synthesis of a common milk component is unlikely. Conceivably a different protein in the milks of other species may serve the purpose that β-lactoglobulin serves in the synthesis of ruminant milks. Alternatively β-lactoglobulin may fill a unique requirement in the nutrition of young ruminants. Attention is drawn to –SH groups which appear to be largely confined to β-lactoglobulin in ruminant milks (see following on whey proteins).

(a) *Milk lipids*. The bulk (99%) of bovine milk lipids exists in the form of fat globules which average 2–3 μ in diameter (Figs. 2 and 3). The remainder occurs in membrane fragments in the skim milk phase. The lipids of milk fat globules are largely (98–99%) glycerides. These lipids also include *ca.* 1% phospholipid, 0.06% glycolipid, 0.30% cholesterol, which is 85–95% in the nonesterified form, and traces of many other lipid classes (free fatty acids, hydrocarbons including carotene, sterols and fat-soluble vitamins). The composition of bovine milk lipids has been very extensively investigated and the knowledge is fairly complete (see Section V). So far as is known, the milk lipids of all mammalian species, as is established for the cow, the human and commonly used experimental animals, occur as globules composed of triglycerides. Similarly, it would be expected that the skim milk phase of milks from all species would contain

---

* See also Addendum on lactose synthetase.

small amounts (0–5% of the total) of lipid in the form of membrane vesicles and fragments, as has been shown for the cow and goat,[291,348] and cellular material (macrophages, sloughed epithelial cells and cell debris).[56,347]

(b) *Casein*. Casein is the name given to a family of milk proteins which comprise about 3.0% of cow's milk. These exist in milk in particles known as casein micelles. Cow's milk contains α-, β-, γ-, and κ-caseins. These vary primarily in phosphorus content (1.0, 0.6, 0.1 and 0.2% respectively) and amino acid composition. A number of genetic variants have been demonstrated for these proteins and κ-casein is unique for the fact that it contains a glycomacropeptide, cleavage of which causes the casein micelles to aggregate in the presence of ionic calcium. This is the basic mechanism of curd formation by action of rennet in cheese making. In cow's milk the "whole" casein contains approximately 60% α-, 25% β-, 5% γ- and 10 to 15% κ-components.

Casein seems to exist characteristically as micelles in all milks. These micelles range from 30 to 300 nm and average about 120 nm in cow's milk. Human milk casein micelles are somewhat smaller in size, but their appearance under the electron microscope is quite similar to those from milks of cow, goat, rat and mouse. Electron photomicrographs (Fig. 13) show bovine casein micelles. Ultrastructural evidence suggests that casein micelles are composed of sub-units of about 15–20 nm in diameter.[55]

Although small amounts of lipid are recovered with casein micelles, they are not lipoproteins. The associated lipid appears to be coincidentally entrained. Small fat globules and/or membrane fragments become trapped in casein prepared either by sedimentation or precipitation.

(c) *Whey proteins*. Although the interest of protein chemists has tended to concentrate on two proteins (β-lactoglobulin and α-lactalbumin) remaining in skim milk on removal of casein, the mixture of proteins present is quite complex, especially if the myriad enzymes[328] are considered. The approximate percentage concentrations in cow's milk of the principal whey proteins are: β-lactoglobulin 0.4, α-lactalbumin 0.1, classical globulins including immune globulins 0.07 and bovine serum albumin 0.03.

β-lactoglobulin (cow) is a simple protein insoluble in dilute salt solutions and existing as a dimer of two identical peptide chains and having a total molecular weight of 36,000 daltons. It contains one –SH group per chain and exists in a number of genetic variants. The heat denaturation of this protein, and protein(s) of the milk fat globule membrane, releases traces of H_2S which imparts a "cooked" or "nutty" flavor to cow's milk.[149]

α-lactalbumin is a simple protein of 16,000 daltons molecular weight. It is the B protein, which together with the A protein, galactosyl transferase, forms the enzyme complex of lactose synthetase.[45,52] α-lactalbumin is unique for its high content (7%) of tryptophan and its structural resemblance to lysozyme.[240]

The immune globulins which are markedly elevated in milk for the first week or so following parturition drop to low levels for the balance of the lactation. These proteins are very important to the newborn ruminant which in comparison to the human infant acquires very little antibody transfer via the placenta and depends substantially on gaining antibodies from milk across the intestinal mucosa. The function, if any, of the classical globulin fraction in mid lactation milk is not known. The subject of the bovine globulins has been reviewed.[57] The importance of the immune globulins and other factors in human milk for host resistance to infection have been presented by

Mata and Wyatt.[231] For further information on immunoglobulin secretion in colostrum, see the report by A. K. Lascelles in ref. 306 and the review by J. E. Butler in ref. 209.

Serum albumin of cow's milk is identical to serum albumin of cow's blood.[240,295] This protein is made in the liver. Whether it is also synthesized by mammary tissue is not known, but the question should be readily resolvable by tracer experiments. Serum albumin binds (carries) fatty acids and is important in the lipid transport system of the circulation,[107] and possibly in mammary tissue.

(d) *Other components.* From the standpoints of synthesis and composition of milk, lactose, the milk salts and ions are significant. The synthesis of lactose has been mentioned in connection with α-lactalbumin in the preceding section on whey proteins. It will be considered further in the context of cell and membrane function. The milk salts are unique for the remarkable levels of calcium that are present and for the fact that the $Na^+ - K^+$ balance tends to resemble that in the cell where the K^+ concentration is elevated as compared to blood in which higher levels of Na^+ exist. This matter is thoroughly reviewed by Linzell and Peaker.[221]

In summary, the synthesis and secretion of milk involves the assembly and transport from the cell of milk fat globules, casein micelles, globulins and simple proteins some of which appear to derive from the blood, lactose, a soluble dissacharide, various ions and water. Coincident to these processes and to some extent essentially for nutrition of the young, a wide array of additional (trace) substances are entrained from the blood and the lactating cell into milk.

C. *General relationship of lipids to lactation*

There are hundreds of species of mammals and these show large variations in milk lipid composition. The ruminants—cow, goat, sheep, deer, etc.—produce a milk fat which is relatively unique for containing substantial amounts of short-chain fatty acids (C_4–C_{12}) esterified in the triglycerides. The fatty acid composition of the milk lipids is not highly responsive to diet. On the other hand, milk lipids of monogastrics such as the human or pig are readily influenced by diet. For example, the amount of linoleate in human milk fat can be markedly increased by feeding corn oil to the mother.[150] The marine mammals (whales, porpoises, and seals) are monogastrics that live on organisms the lipids of which are highly unsaturated (krill and fish). As a result both adipose tissue and milk lipids of these animals are highly unsaturated. Because the energy storage and metabolism of the marine mammals is based primarily on lipid, their milks are very low in carbohydrate (lactose). Some data demonstrating the extremes between species in fatty acid composition of total milk lipids are given in Table 2. We will not know how significant species variations are until more research is conducted on the full spectrum of lactating mammals. At present it is well established that there are wide variations in the levels of fat and in the fatty acid compositions of milk.[155,245] We are led to believe, however, that the mechanisms of synthesis and secretion of milk lipids are generally similar for most mammals.

The functioning of the mammary gland from the standpoint of lipid metabolism involves the following general phenomena: (1) lipolysis of serum lipoprotein lipids and transport of products into the lactating cell; (2) transport of low molecular weight lipid precursors (acetate, β-hydroxybutyrate, $PO_4\equiv$, etc.) from the blood into the

TABLE 2. *Fatty Acid Composition of Milk Lipids from Several Species*[a]

	Human		Cow		
Fatty acid[b]	Fat free diet	Corn oil diet	Summer	Winter	Harp seal
4:0	—	—	3.6	3.5	—
6:0	—	—	1.3	1.4	—
8:0	—	—	0.9	1.1	—
10:0	—	—	2.4	2.7	—
12:0	7.9	3.0	2.7	3.9	0.2
13:0	—	—	0.1	0.1	—
14:0	9.0	2.3	9.8	12.7	5.0
14:1	—	—	—	—	1.1
15:0	—	—	1.1	1.0	—
16:0	23.5	13.1	25.4	34.4	11.8
16:1	6.8	1.4	0.9	1.3	17.7
17:0	—	—	0.7	0.7	—
18:0	3.2	3.0	15.8	11.6	2.3
18:1	36.9	31.4	—	—	26.5
18:1 cis	—	—	24.3	19.9	—
18:1 trans	—	—	6.4	2.5	—
18:2 + 3	7.3	43.0	1.9	1.5	1.1
18:4	—	—	—	—	1.5
20:1	—	—	—	—	4.5
20:4	—	—	—	—	1.0
20:5	—	—	—	—	12.5
22:5	—	—	—	—	3.1
22:6	—	—	—	—	11.9

[a]These data are wt% by gas chromatography of methyl esters and are taken from studies of the human,[150] holstein herd milk fat during summer and winter[282] and a single sample of harp seal milk (S. Patton and M. E. Q. Pilson, unpublished).

[b]Fatty acids are listed: number of carbons colon number of double bonds. For the cow milk fats 18:1 was resolved to *cis* and *trans* isomers.

lactating cell; and (3) the synthesis and assembly of milk lipids within the cell and the secretion of milk lipids from the cell. In order to understand the biochemistry and physiology of lipids in the gland it is helpful to place the foregoing primary phenomena in the context of gland morphology and ultrastructure of the lactating cell.

In recent years it has become a practice to compile and publish papers from scientific symposia. A number of compilations on lactation and related subjects are available[98,289,306] as are reviews and symposium papers related to various aspects of milk lipid synthesis and composition.[48,113,245,338,349]

II. RELATIONSHIP OF GENERAL BODY METABOLISM TO THAT OF THE MAMMARY GLAND

A. General metabolism

Questions concerning metabolism of the mammary gland soon lead to complex considerations of the whole mammal.[72] While we cannot consider total metabolism here in depth, it is important that some sense of whole animal relationships to the functioning of the mammary gland be conveyed to the reader.

The various regulators and metabolites taken up by the mammary gland reach it via the circulation and ultimately through arterial capillaries. The state of the blood at any given time is established by equilibria with every organ and tissue of the body. Of course some sites in the body have more influence than others on the level and state of any given blood component, but the total milieu is determined by a complex of sources. For example, while the lungs are a crucial factor in levels of gases (N_2, O_2, CO_2) in the blood, respiration in every cell of the body is also contributing to the balance. During physical exertion muscle tissue is assuming increased importance in the balance. During lactation the mammary gland becomes much more active not only in exchange of respiratory gases but also in many other interactions with the circulation.

In considering lipid metabolism of the mammary gland the diet provides a logical starting point. Both lipid and non-lipid constituents of food supply some of the metabolic substrates for the gland. Food is broken down in the gut by digestive enzymes acting under appropriate conditions of pH. Bile from the liver, which incidentally is rich in lipids (phospholipids, cholesterol, bile salts), enters the gut and assists in the physical and chemical disintegration of the food. In particular, food fat is emulsified into a fine dispersion and rendered more readily hydrolyzed by lipase. Thus an immediate effect in the gut is a mixing of dietary lipids (exogenous) with bile lipids (endogenous). Principal products of digestion (fatty acids, amino acids, carbohydrates, etc.) are transported into mucosal cells lining the small intestine and from there into the circulation. These mechanisms include mixing and transport of fatty acids, monoglycerides and cholesterol derived from the diet and bile. The lipids entering the intestinal mucosa can be therein directly incorporated into lipoproteins which enter the lymph and eventually the blood at the thoracic duct. Fatty acids of roughly twelve carbons or less enter the portal venous system directly from the mucosa. These are degraded primarily in the liver. The resulting acetate may be used for energy or for synthesis (fatty acids, amino acids, cholesterol, etc.). Carbohydrates of the circulation, such as glucose and fructose, also feed into diverse uses all over the body. These include the generation of acetate for fatty acid synthesis, especially in adipose and mammary tissue, the synthesis of glyceride and phospholipid glycerol via the triose phosphate pathway, production of glycogen, particularly in the liver, and the synthesis of amino acids, particularly glutamic and aspartic acids. Blood glucose is also the substrate used by mammary tissue to synthesize lactose.

The foregoing general relationships are presented in the schemes of Fig. 4. These suffice to show the extensive involvement of mammary tissue with other tissues regarding lipid metabolism. In addition to metabolites, various hormones and enzymes generated in other glands and tissues of the body affect the mammary gland. Development of the lobuloalveolar system of the mammary gland depends on estrogen and progesterone from the ovarian follicle, the corpus luteum and the placenta. Cytodifferentiation of the mammary epithelium to produce milk requires insulin from the pancreas, hydrocortisone from the adrenals and prolactin from the pituitary. Release of milk, so-called "let-down", from the alveoli is produced by contraction of myoepithelial cells under the stimulus of oxytocin, another pituitary hormone. There are species variations in the hormones which influence mammary development and lactation.

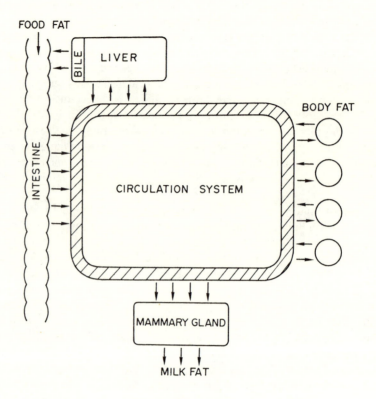
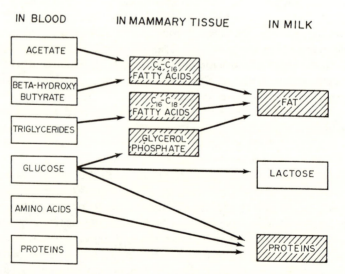

FIG. 4. Upper: Pathways of lipid metabolism in the whole animal that are related to the synthesis of milk lipids. Lower: A scheme denoting the principal substances taken up from the circulation and used by mammary tissue in the synthesis of the major milk components: fat, lactose and protein. (From *Milk*, by S. Patton. Copyright © 1969 by Scientific American Inc. All rights reserved.)

Moreover, the nomenclature and characterization of these hormones is in a state of flux, and considerable overlap in their structure and function exists. The precise modes of action and interaction of hormones in relation to lactation in the intact animal are still difficult to interpret. The subject of hormonal effects on the mammary gland in organ culture has been examined by Forsyth.[103]

The basic chemical transformations of substrates in lipid metabolism are accomplished by enzymes. An incredible number of enzymatic reactions are involved in digesting, synthesizing, transforming, moving, storing and degrading lipids in the animal body. A number of the synthetic pathways and enzymes are discussed subsequently (Section IV) in connection with synthesis of milk lipids. The degradative or lipolytic enzymes include classical lipases which release fatty acids from emulsified glycerides, lipoprotein lipases which accomplish that reaction when the glyceride is contained in a lipoprotein, phospholipases which cleave phospholipids in various ways, esterases which hydrolyze fatty acids from cholesterol and other alcohols, various amidases, glycosidases and other enzymes that break down complex lipids. The lipase of adipose tissue alone involves a very complex system of regulators including insulin, glucagon, epinephrine, catecholamine and cyclic adenosing monophosphate. The lipolytic enzymes are the subject of a review[156] in this series of publications, and in a later more comprehensive exposition.[51]

B. *The rumen*

Closely allied to consideration of diet in relation to mammary function is the rumen. While this remarkable organ is only found in a group of herbivorous mammals (cow, goat, sheep, deer, buffalo, etc.) it is of profound importance in establishing properties of the milk and milk products consumed in vast quantities by humans all over the world. Since rumen function is related to total body metabolism, the organ is involved in the production and properties of meat as well.

What is the rumen? It is a first or fore stomach ahead of the true stomach. In essence it is a large (30 to 60 gallons capacity in the cow) fermentation tank. In a sense there is an analogy between the ruminants and marine organisms. The animals that live in the ocean are surrounded by a nutritional soup. There is a vast plant and animal microbial life which floats freely in the ocean. This is the primary food in the marine environment and is the basis of the food chain which extends up to the sharks and whales. The ruminant encloses its own ocean and with the aid of microorganisms makes its own nutritional soup therein. The crude plant materials it consumes serve as the substrate for and cause of a complex microbial population of bacteria and protozoa that proliferate in its rumen. One-cell plants and animals such as bacteria, protozoa, phytoplankton, zooplankton, etc. are highly nutritious. They usually contain a desirable spectrum of high-quality proteins, minerals and vitamins, plus adequate lipid and carbohydrate for energy purposes. So two important things are accomplished simultaneously in the rumen. One is the production of usable fermentation products, such as acetate, propionate and butyrate, and the second is production of a crop of microbial cells, both on a continuous basis. The cells move with the ingesta to the true stomach where they are digested and utilized as high-quality food.

Because of the influence of Malthus, some have reasoned that the world would reach a point at which animal agriculture could no longer be maintained. People would be in competition with animals for available grain and the animals would have to be eliminated. The research of Virtanen[364] has shown that not only in theory but even in practice this need not be so. Because the ruminant is able to utilize crude cellulosic and fibrous plant materials and simple forms of nitrogen such as urea in generating high-quality nutrients in its rumen, the ruminant does not need to compete with man because man's digestive system cannot derive food value from such materials. So there is a challenge to put ruminant agriculture on an equivalent economic basis throughout the world. Meat and milk from the ruminants are an important basis of the good life in Western culture and these commodities could go a long way in fighting malnutrition and starvation in the rest of the world.

The physiology, cell biology and biochemistry of the rumen is complex. The organisms grow in a complicated symbiosis and very few of them have proven amenable to isolation and study. For extended consideration of the subject, the reader is directed to the text by Hungate[148] and published proceedings from international symposia on ruminant physiology.[216,289] In addition, Viviani[366] has prepared an excellent review of long-chain fatty acid metabolism in the rumen. We will limit our consideration to aspects of rumen metabolism that relate directly to mammary lipid metabolism.

The rumen, while it does effect some oxidative reactions especially within resident microorganisms, is a powerfully anaerobic environment. It generates hydrogen; it produces methane from CO_2; it gives off the strong reducing agent H_2S; and it hydrogenates unsaturated lipids. This latter reaction, often referred to as biohydrogenation, and cellulose hydrolysis are two of the unique biochemical reactions occurring in the rumen. Both appear to be accomplished by –SH-dependent enzymes. Any attempts to emulate *in vitro* the cell biology or biochemistry of the rumen must take into account its very low redox potential and its functional dependence on reduced sulfur compounds.

1. *Volatile fatty acids*

Hexoses from breakdown of cellulose, plant glycolipids, pectins, starches and other plant components are readily fermented by rumen microorganisms. While a great variety of products result, the yields of acetate, propionate and butyrate are important. These acids accumulate in the rumen to a concentration of several moles per liter. They enter the circulation directly through the rumen wall and through the linings of subsequent stomach compartments. Propionate is converted to glycogen in the liver and butyrate is converted to β-hydroxybutyrate primarily in the rumen epithelium and also in the liver. This latter compound together with acetate is removed from the blood by the ruminant mammary gland and both compounds are used in the synthesis of milk lipids, particularly for the short-chain acids that are so characteristic of ruminant milk fat. The subjects of volatile fatty acid production in the rumen is reviewed by Leng and their metabolism in the animal body by Annison and Armstrong in a recent symposium proceedings.[289] This proceedings also contains reviews on lipid metabolism in the rumen by Keeney, on biohydrogenation of dietary fats in ruminants by Dawson and Kemp, and on lipid digestion in the ruminant by Lough.

2. *Microbial lipids*

The research of Katz and Keeney[164,165] on the nature of rumen lipids has established the important role rumen bacteria and protozoa play in contributing unusual fatty

TABLE 3. *Composition of Fatty Acids in Bovine Rumen Digesta and Dietary Hay Lipids*[a]

	Fatty acid (wt. %)												
	14:0Br	14:0	14:1	15:0Br	15:0	16:0Br	16:0	16:1	17:0	18:0	18:1	18:2	18:3
Digesta	0.8	2.3	—	2.8	2.5	1.0	26.6	—	2.6	46.0	7.0	2.8	5.3
Hay	—	0.9	0.8	—	0.8	—	33.9	1.2	—	3.8	3.0	24.0	31.0

[a] Data of Katz and Keeney.[164]

acids to the metabolism of their host. A selection from their data presented in Table 3 shows the profound difference in the fatty acid composition of the rumen digesta as compared with that of lipids in the animal's diet. The digesta, of course, is a mixture of bacteria, protozoa and feed ingredients and from the standpoint of lipid composition the constitutional lipids of the microorganisms and the feed as well as metabolic transformations of feed lipids by the organisms and their enzymes are included. From the standpoint of their constitutional lipids the microorganisms are the source of the fatty acids with branched and odd numbered carbon chains. In fact, as shown by Katz and Keeney, the phosphatidyl ethanolamine fractions from rumen bacteria and protozoa are substantially composed of these acids. They have also shown that the uniqueness of rumen lipids extends to positions of double bonds and oxygenations (carbonyl and hydroxyl groups) in the fatty acids. The ultimate fate of the microbial fatty acids is to enter the general metabolism of the animal in the manner of fatty acids from the feed. As a consequence, microbial fatty acids are not only burned for energy, they are deposited in milk fat and adipose tissue (meat) throughout the body. Of course, on consumption by humans these microbial fatty acids in milk and meat from ruminants enter the human body metabolic pathways. It is a conservative estimate that cow's milk fat contains at least 10% fatty acids of microbial origin.

3. Biohydrogenation

A profound difference in fatty acid composition of lipids from dietary hay and rumen digesta, presented in Table 3, concerns the C18 acids. The hay lipids, as is characteristic of lipids from green plants in general, are rich in linoleate and linolenate. These are virtually absent from the rumen digesta, whereas it contains much stearic acid. The cause of this difference, as discovered by Reiser,[303] is hydrogenation. A complex of biochemical reactions brought about by the rumen microorganisms converts the abundant C18 unsaturated fatty acids in ruminant feeds to stearic acid primarily and small amounts of *trans* octadec-11-enoic acid, so called vaccenic acid and related enoic isomers. This establishes the distinctive role of stearic acid in ruminant lipid metabolism and emphasizes the profound relevance of rumen action to any consideration of dietary lipids in ruminants.

The definitive work from Tove's laboratory,[181,310] using the rumen organism *Butyrivibrio fibrosolvens* in pure culture and as a source of essential enzymes, has shed much light on the biochemical mechanisms involved in biohydrogenation of fatty acids, particularly linoleic and linolenic acids. In order to be hydrogenated, the appropriate acids must be unesterified,[114,132,276] the enzyme in question apparently requiring a free carboxyl group.[181] While some linoleate is synthesized by rumen organisms[266] and some linoleate and linolenate escapes hydrogenation in the form of constitutional lipid in protozoa, the proportion is small and of the order of a few percent. However, it must be of indispensable importance in meeting the essential fatty acid requirement of the ruminant.

Katz and Keeney[165] have shown that the 2-position in the glycerolphosphatides of rumen holotrich protozoa contains substantial octadecadienoic and octadecatrienoic acids. Presumably these are the *cis* 9,12 and *cis* 9,12,15 isomers, the former being capable of meeting the animal's essential fatty acid needs including substrate requirement for prostaglandin synthesis. So far as is known, the ruminant has no capacity (outside of the rumen) to synthesize linoleate so that despite the intensive reducing conditions in the rumen and the highly effective hydrogenation of dietary linoleate, a path to assure the animal a supply of this essential acid is maintained. This path seems to be at least in part a matter of synthesis of linoleate within protozoa of the rumen and their passage to the true stomach where they yield their linoleate on being digested. It is possible that the unsaturated acids of the protozoa may be assimilated from the feed material, but rumen synthesis of linoleate now seems well documented. In any event, definitive research on the origin of that reaching the true stomach is needed.

4. *Polyunsaturation of milk fat*

A number of consequences follow from the highly saturated nature of the lipids reaching the true stomach in the ruminant, especially in respect to milk lipids. The animal cannot compose functional membranes or synthesize and deposit storage triglycerides using mainly palmitic and stearic acids. In the case of milk fat, short-chain fatty acids (C_4 to C_{12}) are employed to give liquidity at body temperature to triglycerides. Also for melting properties in assembling triglycerides into milk fat globules as well as for membranes and other lipid storage conditions the functioning of the enzyme, stearyl desaturase, is of utmost importance. This enzyme, located in various tissues including those of liver and mammary gland, converts stearic acid to oleic acid and makes the latter widely available in the body. Linoleate tends to be conserved in structural lipids of the ruminant. The ratio of stearic to oleic acid being taken up from the blood by the mammary gland is approximately 2.5:1. In milk fat the ratio is just the reverse due to the action of stearyl desaturase in mammary tissue. A second consequence of the highly saturated fatty acids issuing from the rumen is that ruminant meat and milk fats are relatively saturated. The concern regarding saturated dietary fats in relation to human heart disease has been so great that the feasibility of avoiding hydrogenation in the rumen has been investigated and demonstrated. Scott *et al.*[323,324] have shown that seed oils rich in linoleate can be emulsified into sodium caseinate solution, spray dried and treated with formalin to yield a powder which when fed will resist rumen hydrogenation of the lipid. On movement to the true stomach the protein is hydrolyzed which releases the polyunsaturated lipid, making it available for digestion and assimilation. Using this technique the Australian group has produced milks with fat containing as much as 40% linoleic acid. Bitman *et al.*[32,293] have confirmed these findings and revealed that a "protected" feed product made with safflower oil transfers polyunsaturated acids to milk fat much more effectively than one containing soybean oil.

The practicalities of this *in vitro* route to "polyunsaturated" milk are somewhat open to question. Milk fat as normally produced by the cow is a highly palatable item and non-injurious to health if consumed in reasonable quantities and balanced with some unsaturated fats in other aspects of the diet. Not only in milk but in butter, cream and ice cream, milk fat imparts excellent flavor qualities for which the consumer is willing to pay a fair price. If it is a matter of rendering milk "polyunsaturated", why not add the relatively inexpensive and readily available polyunsaturated oils to the milk as needed? In our experience, milk and milk products containing polyunsaturated oils will have serious flavor problems because such lipids are far more sensitive than normal milk lipids to chemical changes induced by heat, light, air, trace metals, etc. The attribute which distinguishes the flavor of milk and many of its products is blandness of flavor. Even without the keeping quality problem of polyunsaturated fats, it has proven almost impossible to produce a dry whole milk with satisfactory flavor properties because of the ease with which faint off-flavors are perceived in milk. Very possibly for reasons of health considerations, some substantial market may exist for a milk containing a naturally produced polyunsaturated milk fat. Some customers may indeed be willing to pay the additional cost and accept the limitations of such a product and we are indebted to the Australian and US scientists who have shown that the process is commercially feasible. Further information, including fatty acid composition, of so-called protected milk is given in Section V.

Some of the unique unsaturated fatty acids in rumen contents are intermediates or minor by-products of the hydrogenation of polyunsaturated fatty acids in the diet.[164,181]

5. *Unusual fatty acids*

In addition to the unusual odd carbon numbered and branched chain fatty acids that are constitutional in the microflora of the rumen (see data for rumen digesta Table 3), exotic fatty acids are produced by action of the microorganisms on feed components. One of these is phytanic acid.[270] Phytol (1) hydrolyzed from chlorophyll is hydrogenated to dihydrophytol (2) which is then oxidized to the acid (3).

$$CH_3\text{-}CH(CH_3)\text{-}CH_2\text{-}CH_2\text{-}CH_2\text{-}CH(CH_3)\text{-}CH_2\text{-}CH_2\text{-}CH_2\text{-}CH(CH_3)\text{-}CH_2\text{-}CH_2\text{-}C(CH_3)\text{=}CH\text{-}CH_2OH \quad (1)$$

$$CH_3\text{-}CH(CH_3)\text{-}CH_2\text{-}CH_2\text{-}CH_2\text{-}CH(CH_3)\text{-}CH_2\text{-}CH_2\text{-}CH_2\text{-}CH(CH_3)\text{-}CH_2\text{-}CH_2\text{-}CH(CH_3)\text{-}CH_2\text{-}CH_2OH \quad (2)$$

$$CH_3\text{-}CH(CH_3)\text{-}CH_2\text{-}CH_2\text{-}CH_2\text{-}CH(CH_3)\text{-}CH_2\text{-}CH_2\text{-}CH_2\text{-}CH(CH_3)\text{-}CH_2\text{-}CH_2\text{-}CH(CH_3)\text{-}CH_2\text{-}C(\text{=}O)\text{-}OH \quad (3)$$

Phytanic acid together with a number of other unusual fatty acids from the rumen occur in trace amounts in milk fat (see Section V). This acid is notable for its accumulation in Refsum's disease, a rare inborn error of metabolism involving the inability of an individual to initiate oxidation of the molecule.[195] As a consequence, phytanic acid accumulates in organs and tissues of the body in this disease. The condition is particularly detrimental to nerve function and progressively destroys vision and coordination leading to premature death. The biochemistry and physiology of Refsum's disease have been reviewed.[93,346] From complex considerations of the molecular stereochemistry, Lough[223] concludes that phytanic acid from the liver of Refsum's patients could derive from phytanic acid in dairy products among other possible sources.

Two other rumen acids are interesting in light of their derivation and because they do not enter the general lipid metabolism of the body. These are phenylacetic and 3-phenylpropionic acids derived from phenylalanine and tyrosine.[277] These acids contribute to the strong malodor of rumen ingesta. The fact that amino acids are degraded to form these compounds demonstrates the preference of the bacteria to synthesize their own amino acids. This is also reflected in the ruminant's ability to get along without dietary protein and to utilize urea as a sole source of nitrogen.

In summary, certain unique principles need to be borne in mind regarding lipid metabolism in the ruminant. The flow of ingesta from the rumen to the lower alimentary tract is a more or less continuous process and completely different from the meal eating regimen of the monogastric animal. Normally the ruminant never releases a large amount of neutral fat at a given time into the intestine. Rather there is a continuous flow of material containing relatively low levels of lipid mainly in the form of free fatty acids (stearic and palmitic) bound to feed particles and with lesser amounts of mixed lipids contained in bacteria and protozoa. Additional unique aspects of the rumen metabolism are its generation of volatile fatty acids (C_2, C_3, C_4), hydrogenated dietary fatty acids (primarily stearic) and unique microbial fatty acids all of which directly or indirectly become involved in lipid metabolism of the lactating mammary gland.

C. *The serum lipoproteins*

1. *Composition and metabolism*

The basic function of the lipoprotein in the blood serum is to transport lipids to and from the various tissues and organs of the body. This is one of the most active, complicated and challenging areas of biomedical research today. A principal reason for this research activity is the relevance of the subject to human health problems, particularly obesity and heart disease. As a consequence the research is well funded and the information being generated is copious, but the emerging picture of the serum lipoproteins is one of expanding complexity. When we consider that these particles interact with each other and with tissues and organs throughout the body the problem of comprehending their metabolisms is evident. Part of the difficulty may arise from use of radioactive tracers to study the metabolism of the lipoproteins. This gives a picture which while true is a dynamic one, one that derives from many kinds of transfer interactions. Reviews[109,119,253,318] assist in orienting one to the available information on structure and function of the serum lipoproteins.

TABLE 4. *The Composition of Human Serum Lipoprotein Ultracentrifugal Fractions according to Bragdon et al.[40] and Forte et al.[104]* (Data compiled by B. C. Raphael)

Lipoprotein class	Density ρ	Protein	Lipid	TG	PL	CE	UC	Size (Å)
				%				
Chylomicron	< 0.94	2.1	97.9	81.2	7.0	6.4	3.2	1000–5000
VLDL	< 1.019	7.1	92.9	51.8	17.9	16.2	6.0	300–1000
LDL	1.019–1.063	20.7	79.3	9.3	23.1	39.4	7.5	150–300
HDL	1.063–1.210	46.4	53.6	8.1	26.1	17.4	2.0	70–150

Abbreviations: VLDL – very low density lipoprotein; LDL – low density lipoprotein; HDL – high density lipoprotein; TG – triglyceride; PL – phospholipid; CE – cholesterol ester; UC – unesterified cholesterol.

As with many naturally occurring populations, methods of classifying the serum lipoproteins are somewhat arbitrary. One of the most useful and the one employed here is according to density. Another is by electrophoretic mobility. A characterization of the human serum lipoproteins based on data by Bragdon *et al.*[40] and Forte *et al.*[104] is given in Table 4. The latter group provides detail on size and ultrastructure. It will be seen that the size of the serum lipoprotein particles is positively correlated with their lipid contents and negatively related to the amounts of protein they contain. In addition the larger particles, chylomicrons and very low density lipoproteins (VLDLs), are rich in triglycerides, whereas the low density lipoproteins (LDLs) and high density lipoproteins (HDLs) contain relatively greater proportions of their lipids as phospholipids and cholesterol esters. The chylomicrons are elevated in the blood following eating, particularly after a fatty meal and their size is such that they make serum appear opalescent or milky. Properties of chylomicrons from dog, rat and man have been extensively investigated by Zilversmit.[386,387] In agarose or polyacrylamide gel electrophoresis the serum lipoproteins move in the order HDL⟩ LDL⟩VLDL. These are approximately comparable respectively to α-, β- and pre-β-lipoprotein designations used in electrophoresis. Chylomicrons do not move from the origin in electrophoresis. This behavior is plausible. As the serum lipoproteins increase in size they would be expected to move through the gel matrix less rapidly, and coincidentally the larger they are the more neutral lipid and the less charged material (protein and phospholipid) they contain with which to respond to the applied potential.

The knowledge of the origin of serum lipoproteins at present appears to be as follows: It is well known and widely accepted that chylomicrons are formed in the intestinal mucosa. They are secreted there into the lymph and enter the circulation at the thoracic duct. Normally about 15 min is required for the clearing of a chylomicron from the circulation. VLDLs appear to be synthesized in two locations, the intestinal mucosa and the liver.[259] However, the relative amounts that are synthesized at the two sites in any given species is quite uncertain in light of the limited information available. Regarding VLDL synthesis, the liver and mammary gland present an interesting contrast at the cellular level with respect to the anabolism of neutral lipid. The principal triglyceride-bearing product of the hepatocyte is the VLDL, that of the mammary cell the milk fat globule. The milk fat globule is several microns in diameter and >95% triglyceride. The VLDL is about 50% triglyceride and about 0.03–0.1 microns in diameter. The endoplasmic reticulum is the site of triglyceride synthesis in both instances[343,344] and the fatty acid synthetase of liver and mammary tissue appears to be identical.[339] The principal difference is that VLDLs are secreted from the hepatocyte by way of Golgi vesicles,[343] whereas the milk fat globule is secreted by direct envelopment in and expulsion from the plasma membrane (see Section III). The crucial point of departure seems to be that triglycerides are vectored into the cysternae of the endoplasmic reticulum where they can be conducted to the Golgi apparatus in the liver cell, whereas in the mammary cell the triglycerides are retained apparently on the cytoplasmic side of the endoplasmic reticulum. Orotic acid administration is known to produce liver triglyceride accumulation (fatty liver) in the rat. The mode of action involves a block in the movement of VLDLs within the cysternae of the endoplasmic reticulum.[256] Orotic acid levels are remarkably high in the fat-free portion of cow's milk (approximately 0.100 mg/ml),[62] which phase is secreted by way of Golgi vesicles. This evidence indicates that orotic acid is involved in mechanisms of triglyceride accumulation and secretion from the cell.

It is now generally held that VLDL is precursor of LDL. A number of studies[28,90,91] have shown that the proteins of VLDL move to the LDL class. This is what would be predicted on the removal of triglyceride from the VLDL at various sites,[28] including the lactating mammary gland. The origin of HDL is uncertain. There appear to be rather complex relationships among the proteins of the various serum lipoproteins. Windmueller et al.[377] and Eisenberg and Rachmilewitz[91] have recently investigated these relationships in the rat.

There are other lipid-bearing entities in the serum in addition to the classical lipoproteins. One of these is serum albumin, which reversibly binds free fatty acids.[107] The retinol-bearing protein[252] of the blood is an example of a highly specific vehicle for lipid. Because of the ease of labeling serum albumin with fatty acid or more simply injecting fatty acids directly into the blood stream, there is a substantial amount of information on uptake of free fatty acid by various organs of the body. This is somewhat misleading in that there is usually no basis of comparison, for example with triglyceride fatty acid in chylomicrons or VLDLs. Labeling the various serum lipoproteins with individual radioactive lipids in a physiologically acceptable manner is complicated and troublesome. Theoretically, labeling the serum lipoproteins by injection of a radioactive tracer in one animal, isolating the particular lipoprotein and injecting it into a second animal is a desirable approach although dilution of activity in two whole bodies is a problem. Much of the research on lipid metabolism of the heart has utilized free fatty acid, but there seems to be no reason to believe that serum triglycerides may not be equally, if not more important, than serum free fatty acids in the lipid metabolism of this organ.

While Evans et al.[96] demonstrated some years ago that HDLs (alpha-lipoproteins) are the principal lipoproteins in cow's blood and that serum triglycerides were concentrated in a lower density fraction ($\rho < 1.063$), there have been no detailed studies of any species regarding serum lipoprotein during lactation and dry periods until that recently by Raphael et al. They analyzed the serum lipoproteins of the bovine during gestation and lactation by preparative ultracentrifugation[301] and gel electrophoresis.[302] Their studies are significant since it is well established that a substantial

TABLE 5. *Composition and Concentration of Lipids Associated with the Various Bovine Serum Lipoproteins during Lactation.*[a]

Lipoprotein class	Animals no.	Lipid (mg/100ml) of serum	TG	PL	CE	UC
				%		
VLDL	10	4.7 ± 1.9	57	16	22	6.0
LDL	6	35 ± 22	12	28	46	14.
HDL₁	6	162 ± 18	b	44 ± 8.3	49 ± 12.1	10.5 ± 0.0
HDL	6	327 ± 86	b	43 ± 2.8	54 ± 1.6	5.8 ± 4.0

Abbreviations: see Table 4.
[a] Data of Raphael et al.[301] VLDL data are for 0 to 10th week in lactation, for the other classes 5th to 10th week.
[b] Triglycerides not detectable in samples.

fraction of bovine milk fat is derived from fatty acids of serum triglycerides (see following discussion). As might be expected, the cow has relatively low levels of serum lipids. It normally consumes only modest levels of lipid and because of its multiple stomach arrangement the movement of digesta into the small intestine is more gradual and continuous than in meal eating monogastrics such as the human. The latter have surges of food of substantial fat content and this leads to the well-known post-prandial serum lipemia due to chylomicrons released into the blood. Raphael et al. as well as other investigators have noted the relative lack of chylomicrons in cow's blood. They observed serum lipids to range generally from 0.3 to 0.5%; HDLs accounted for 57–76% of the serum lipids and VLDLs for less than 5% in dry animals and on average about 1% in lactating animals. Because the cow in comparison to the human has HDL in the LDL fraction (i.e. $\rho < 1.063$), Raphael et al. subdivided the HDL fraction into HDL (ρ 1.063–1.210) and HDL₁ (ρ 1.040–1.063). Table 5 summarizes some of their data for the lactating cow.

2. Contribution to milk lipids

It has been known for some time that serum triglycerides contribute fatty acids for the synthesis of milk lipids, particularly for triglycerides of the milk fat globules. The initial evidence was provided by arterio-venous differences across the lactating gland of the goat[17] and this has been confirmed with radioactive tracer experiments.[8,31,116,373] It is variously estimated that 20–80% of milk fatty acids and perhaps a mean of about 50% in the cow or goat are derived from serum triglycerides. No doubt the availability of serum lipids for milk lipid synthesis may vary considerably depending upon the nutrition and metabolic state of the animal. The radioactive tracer studies of Glascock et al.[116] and Bishop et al.[31] clearly establish that the serum lipoproteins, especially chylomicrons and low density lipoproteins, are the particular sources of the serum triglycerides used in milkfat synthesis. While chylomicrons as well as VLDLs may be involved in monogastric animals, the study by Raphael et al. presents evidence that in ruminants it is primarily the VLDL fraction that is supplying the triglycerides utilized in milk lipid synthesis. In contrast to the findings of Evans et al.[96] and Raphael et al.[301] Bickerstaffe reports observing significant quantities of chylomicrons in serum of the lactating bovine. Further, he finds triglycerides associated with all of his serum lipoprotein fractions and that all of these are a source of triglyceride fatty acids for contribution to milk triglyceride synthesis (see ref. 98). We suggest that these variations in findings are not actually in conflict, but result from differences in the methods of defining and preparing the serum lipoprotein fractions.

The uptake of serum triglycerides by the mammary gland appears to depend on the action of lipoprotein lipase. This enzyme, which hydrolyzes fatty acids from triglycerides of lipoproteins, is known to increase dramatically in activity in the mammary gland about the time of parturition.[233,307] Of course, the mammary gland is not the only site of lipoprotein lipase in the body. Adipose tissue in particular and many other organs and tissues throughout the body contain this enzyme.[51] It is not clear how the activities in these locations are regulated. Specific peptides associated with the HDL class have been shown to activate lipoprotein lipase.[131,208] Emery[94] reports that lipoproteins vary in their preference for the lipoprotein lipases of various tissues such as adipose and mammary. He suggests further that prolactin may activate lipoprotein lipase of mammary gland and that insulin may be required for the enzyme to function in adipose tissue.* This may need to be evaluated in light of the observations that normal milk is secreted by the cow and goat despite suppression of prolactin release from the pituitary with the drug ergocryptine.[129,319]

Lipolytic action on serum lipoproteins is a significant consideration in many tissues. Schoefl and French[320] have presented graphic evidence of this process in mouse mammary tissue. This has been confirmed by Scow et al.[325] who have postulated a generalized mechanism involving vesicle formation for conveyance of released fatty acids across the endothelium to receptor cells. There is yet much to learn about this process. A consideration of the ultrastructure in this area of mammary tissue suggests some of the problems which further research will encounter. Milk precursors from blood must enter the capillary endothelial cell, move through and out of it into intercellular space. Fluid in this space apparently is continuous with the lymph system, which is known to contain lipids and to drain from the gland. Adipose cells, particularly in some species such as the rat, are in metabolic equilibrium with this intercellular fluid as are alveoli of mammary epithelial cells. Histochemistry and autoradiography coupled with microscopy may help to shed light on this presently obscure area of transport and metabolism. The movement of small water-soluble molecules from the blood into the lactating cell represents a somewhat different transport dilemma than large lipid molecules.

If the lipoproteins are interacting with the endothelial cells lining the capillaries to an extent that chylomicron and VLDL triglycerides are digested, one wonders about other lipids associated with these moieties. Do they exchange with the endothelium membranes? Is this the route by which cholesterol from the diet and in the blood gets into milk? Could this be a preliminary aspect of the mechanism that infilters arterial linings with cholesterol in atherosclerosis? Recently completed experiments at our laboratory indicates that in the fasted rat, all three serum lipoproteins, VLDLs, LDLs and HDLs, are sources of cholesterol that gains entry to milk. These experiments are discussed in connection with synthesis of milk lipids (Section IV). Also discussed in that section is the controversy which centers on whether serum triglycerides yield monoglycerides additionally or only free fatty acids and glycerol as a result of lipoprotein lipase action in mammary tissue. The acylation of monoglyceride derived

---

* See also Addendum literature on prolactin and lipoprotein lipase.

in the intestinal lumen by action of pancreatic lipase on dietary triglycerides is a documented path of triglyceride synthesis in intestinal mucosa and adipose tissue.[147,294,327]

Because no appreciable arterio-venous difference could be detected across the mammary gland for free fatty acid, it has been thought until recently that they are not used. Radioactive tracer data obtained by Annison et al.[8] indicate that the situation is obscured by fatty acid exchange reactions in which free fatty acids are entering the tissue from arterial blood and reappearing in venous blood in the form of triglycerides. Thus some significant fraction of blood lipid taken up by the mammary gland appears to be in the form of free fatty acid. One estimate is one-fifth.[94]

Again on the basis of arterio-venous differences it is held that serum phospholipids do not contribute to milk lipids. But it is pointed out by Easter et al.[88] that serum phospholipids could be contributing to milk phospholipids to a significant degree without producing a detectable arterio-venous difference. This is because the serum phospholipid pool is large and that in the milk small. The evidence from their study as well as that of Annison et al.[8] is that milk phospholipids are synthesized *de novo* in mammary tissue.

The milk lipids of the bovine are yellow due to the presence of β-carotene and generally the Jersey and Guernsey breeds produce milk lipids with more carotene than other breeds such as the Holstein which breed is the origin of about 85% of the milk in the United States. Goats, and most other ruminants, have carotene-free milk lipids. The carotene in cow's milk fat is of dietary origin and goats generally have diets very similar to those of cows. The implication is a difference in metabolism of carotene by the two species. The relative difference in milk carotene among breeds of dairy cows has been attributed to a difference in the conversion of carotene to vitamin A in the intestinal mucosa. We have noted in the course of our research that both the serum lipoproteins and the mammary tissue lipids from the cow are rich in carotene. Destruction or non-absorption of carotene in the goat are possibilities. In an exploratory experiment we injected 60 mg of a water-dispersable β-carotene into the jugular vein of a lactating goat. Milk was collected twice a day for 10 days and the lipids extracted from all the samples. There was never any evidence of carotene transport into the milk. It was estimated that the amount of carotene injected was sufficient to impart a hue of the intensity of orange juice to the total blood volume of the animal. Experiments of this type will bear repeating in various ways, of course, but we find the species difference intriguing. Another interesting metabolic path to explore is that of carotene through the lactating cell. As compared with total globule lipid, membranes of the milk fat globule are enriched in carotene.[53] Carotene may prove to be a useful indicator of how lipophilic molecules behave in cell membranes *in vivo*.

D. *Depressed milk fat*

A rather mystifying aberration of lipid metabolism in the lactating cow is the so-called low milk fat syndrome. The substantial research on this problem has been reviewed[71] and reveals a complex of factors involving total lipid metabolism of the animal. The difficulty is usually encountered in high producing animals on a high concentrate–low roughage diet. More particularly abundance of highly digestible carbohydrate and absence of fibrous matter in the diet are conducive. The level of fat in the milk may drop from a mean of 4% to as low as 1% and of course this is of profound economic importance.

A remarkable feature of the syndrome is that at the same time the fat is not being secreted in the milk it tends to be more readily deposited in adipose tissue so that metabolic regulation affecting the whole animal is involved. The availability of serum triglyceride fatty acids to various tissues and organs of the body is dependent upon lipoprotein lipase. In this connection Schotz and Garfinkel[321] have shown that lipoprotein lipases at various sites show different degrees of activity depending on the nutritional state of the animal. Perhaps the most attractive explanation is the glucogenic theory which states that milk fat depression involves increased uptake and decreased release of fatty acids from adipose tissue due to elevated serum glucose and insulin. The latter activates adipose lipoprotein lipase.

III. STRUCTURE AND FUNCTION OF MAMMARY EPITHELIUM

A. *General features of the mammary gland*

There is much variation in the appearance of the mammary glands among the mammalian species. The marine mammals (seals, porpoises, whales, etc.) are generally streamlined animals with two bilateral glands smoothly imbedded in adipose tissue in the mid-ventral region. The only overt evidence of the glands are slits through which the nipples project on nursing stimulus of the young. Glands of the kangaroo appear to involve milks of different composition, including lipids, being given at different locations in relation to the age of the young.[120] The duckbill platypus does not appear to have true nipples but instead hairy spots on the skin which are dampened by secreted milk. In the rat, the mammary glands with multiple bilateral nipples extend from the body junctures of the hind legs to those of the front legs and into the neck region. The domestic cow which has been bred toward a huge mammary gland has four teats (nipples) while the goat has two. The human and bovine exhibit decided gross differences in mammary gland appearance, the actual mammary structure and function for the two are comparable. The nipple in the human is in essence the bovine teat and the mass of one human mammary gland is analogous to a quarter of the bovine udder. In contrast to the ducts leading to a rather large cistern in the cow, a series of ducts lead directly to the outer surface of the human nipple. But at the level of ducts and alveoli the appearances of the two mammary glands are quite similar. Electron photomicrographs of human lactating tissue have recently been published (see Addendum, Tobon and Salazar) and its ultrastructure closely resembles that of other species. Human casein micelles and milk fat globules appear typical. The apppearance of bovine tissue at various scale levels is presented schematically in Fig. 5. Excluding that for the gross gland (Fig. 5a), the schemes for the tissue (Fig. 5b), the alveolus (Fig. 5c) and the cell (Fig. 5d) are broadly representative across mammalian species. Perhaps the only substantial species variable is the amount of adipose tissue and cells distributed in the gland (see following).

The composition of mammary tissue regarding the kinds of tissues, cells and structures involved is a highly significant consideration in attempts to understand the bio-

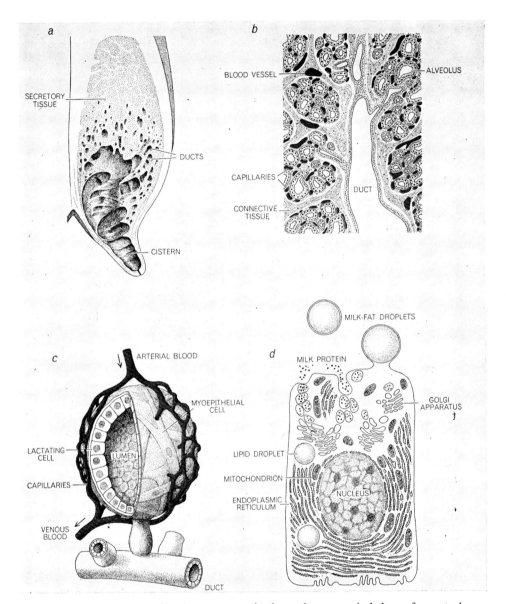

FIG. 5. The appearance of bovine mammary gland at scales progressively larger from a to d. (a) cross-section of one udder quarter, (b) structure with a small section of tissue showing groups of alveoli, capillaries, a large duct, etc., (c) structure of a single alveolus showing arrangement of lactating cells and (hollow) lumen area into which milk is secreted, (d) a scheme of the lactating mammary cell illustrating the mechanisms of protein and fat secretion and showing the principal membrane systems of the cell, i.e., endoplasmic reticulum, mitochondrial, Golgi apparatus and plasma membrane (cell envelope). (From *Milk*, by S. Patton. Copyright © 1969 by Scientific American Inc. All rights reserved.)

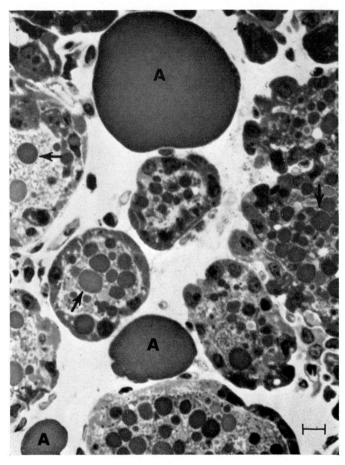

FIG. 6. Lactating mammary tissue of the rat. Adipose cells (A) are evident in space between alveoli. Numerous secreted milk fat globules (arrows) ranging up to 10 μ in diameter are present within lumens of alveoli. Bar (lower right) represents 10 μ. (Photomicrograph courtesy of B. H. Stemberger.)

chemistry and physiology of the gland. Unfortunately there are few quantitative data available. Snipes and Lengemann[341] present an analysis of lactating guinea pig mammary tissue. Excluding milk, they find 55.7% secretory epithelium, 39.8% supportive tissue and 4.5% blood plasma. While these data make supportive tissue a catch-all category, the study suggests the need for more extensive analysis particularly with respect to species differences.

1. *Adipose tissue*

One of the reasons that further characterization of mammary tissue is needed is to define what role adipose tissue may play in the functioning of the lactating mammary gland. Moreover, it is obvious that a substantial portion (39.8%) of the lactating gland tissue in the guinea pig is not directly involved in the synthesis of milk but may be indirectly important in storage and/or transport mechanism from the circulation to the alveoli. In examining the structure of mammary tissue with the light microscope we note that cow and goat tissues exhibit mainly alveoli which rather closely abut one another without extensive quantities of intervening tissue. It is true that layers of adipose tissue next to the skin and between the gland and the abdominal wall are usually encountered in these species, but a heavy interspersion of adipose cells between alveoli is not. However, with the rat there frequently are areas of secretory epithelium in which adipose tissue cells occupy interalveolar space (Fig. 6). Whether these cells bear any relationship to lipid metabolism of the mammary epithelial cell is not known. In considering the variables that might influence the milk fat contents among species, the level of lipids in the blood and the lipogenic capabilities of the mammary epithelium are two obvious factors. However, some of the species variations may relate to the capacity of the gland to maintain and use adipose stores. The blubber of marine mammals and the high fat content of their milks may be related in this way. As discussed elsewhere, the ruminants exhibit very modest levels of blood lipids. Mainly this is a result of their consuming diets relatively low in fat. However, in the case of lactating ruminants, lipid is further reduced in the body by the drain of synthesis and secretion of milk. As a consequence one normally does not observe infiltration of ruminant mammary epithelium with adipose deposits. It is of interest to note in a study by Stewart[347] in which a lipid emulsion was intravenously infused into a lactating (Jersey) cow, that heavily laden adipose cells were found in the mammary interalveolar spaces. This condition very much resembled that which we noted in lactating rat mammary tissue and suggests that both species and dietary factors are involved.

It is reasonable to assume that in some species, possibly including the human, adipose cells intimately dispersed between lactating alveoli are involved in metabolism of the mammary epithelium and thus in the synthesis of milk. The flux of fatty acids into and out of these adipose cells will relate to some of the same capillary bed and interalveolar space that is serving the mammary epithelium. However, it will require inspired research to prove this assumption. One of the most logical approaches would be to demonstrate that fatty acids held in the adipose cells eventually are incorporated into milk fat. An initial difficulty would be to separate adipose cells, milk fat globules and fat droplets (formative milk fat globules) within mammary epithelial cells. These are all very low density particles with very high triglyceride contents. Some problems involved in characterizing the intracellular lipid droplets have been described[140] (see also p. 42). In theory, microscopy-autoradiography should be able to provide evidence of movement of a labeled lipid from an adipose cell into a milk fat droplet. This would depend on exhausting any other source of the label in the body—a rather unlikely possibility since labeling of adipose lipids would probably have occurred all over the body. Moreover, microscopy-autoradiography in addition to being a sophisticated scientific technique is a demanding art-form. Perhaps one might be able to supply the evidence with this technique if it were suitably applied to a mammary gland system first labeled with a tracer lipid and then perfused with unlabeled blood. A time sequence then might suggest that photographic grains (tracer fatty acid) moved from adipose cell to intercellular space, to secretory cell, to intracellular fat droplet and finally to milk fat globule.

In any event the amount of adipose tissue in mammary gland and its importance in lactation needs to be investigated. When one thinks of the large number of studies conducted on homogenates and cell preparations from mammary tissue and when one considers that as much as 40% of the tissue is not of a cell type or structural material involved directly with milk synthesis and secretion, it becomes clear that the meaning of many published experimental results may be nebulous indeed. Judged in this light, the mammary tissue homogenate and the so-called microsomal pellet are experimental systems with serious limitations. Obviously if they include adipose cells or their fragments one can say with certainty that radio tracer experiments using such systems may yield confounded results. A means of isolating lactating alveoli to facilitate metabolic studies has been developed (see Addendum, Katz et al.).

B. *The alveolus*

The fundamentally important unit of structure in the mammary gland is a micro-organ known as an alveolus (see Figs. 5c and 6). There are vast numbers of these connected by a system of ducts which enable the milk output from an individual lactating cell to be pooled with that from millions of other cells. The alveolus is a hollow sphere-like arrangement of mammary epithelial cells. The cells are a continuous monolayer and at some point on the sphere they lead away to form a connection to the duct system. The hollow central areas of the alveolus is known as the lumen and it holds the milk secreted from the cells. Myoepithelial cells stretch across the exterior surface of the alveolus and these may be stimulated to contract by the hormone, oxytocin, thus compressing the alveolus and forcing milk from its lumen into the duct system. Oxytocin is released from the pituitary and reaches the mammary tissue by the circulation. Its release is stimulated by sucking or massage of the gland. In experimental work it is sometimes necessary to administer oxytocin in order to obtain milk from an intractable animal (such as a sow) or to obtain residual or very freshly secreted milk from a gland. The effect of the hormone can be very dramatic. Upon administration of oxytocin to some large animals, milk freely streams from the gland and one must literally catch it in a pan or bucket. Use of about 0.1 USP units of oxytocin administered intramuscularly is helpful in collecting milk from laboratory rats.

The alveolus is nourished by capillary blood flow to and from its exterior surface. Presumably it is also bathed in lymph and lymph may be conceived as filling intra-cellular space between endothelial cells of the capillaries and lactating epithelial cells of the alveolus. It seems probable that the tissue has rather complex equilibria regarding flow of metabolites. Generally this flow of metabolites would be into the lactating cells and the relative movement of metabolites in the lymph system is conceived as lagging in relation to uptake from the blood into these cells. However, back flow of constituents from milk to blood does occur, especially when removal of milk from the gland is delayed. No doubt many variables enter into this system and it becomes complex indeed when one considers that a number of cell types in addition to the lactating cells may be involved. The possibilities that the capillary bed may collapse, that cells may have rest periods and that cyclic phenomena may be involved are additional considerations. But in considering blood lipids as precursors of milk lipids, and in attempting to conceptualize the transport and other molecular mechanisms involved, one has to visualize some type of structural-functional pathway out of the blood into the cell. This is considered further in Section IV dealing with synthesis of milk lipids.

The alveolar structure imposes on the lactating cell an asymmetry. The basal side of the cell is oriented toward interalveolar space, lymph and circulation. The apical side of the cell faces the lumen and the lateral sides are oriented against adjacent cells. It is of interest then to note that isolation of plasma membrane from the mammary epithelium will involve membrane with three different structural-functional states. That in the basal area involves primarily transport of metabolites into the cell; the apical membrane is concerned with milk secretion and the lateral membrane is concerned with cell–cell interactions and communications. No doubt these are three different membranes, although they may tend to equilibrate with each other if a fluid situation in the membrane maintains as suggested by Singer and Nicolson[335] among others. In all probability, the tight junctions which occur in the apical intersecting regions between cells prevent equilibrium of membrane constituents at the secretory end with those of lateral membranes. It is claimed that Na^+, K^+-ATPase is absent from the apical membrane but occurs in the rest of the plasma membrane of the lactating cell.[194]

Binucleated cells and cells with apparent cytoplasmic bridges or openings (holes) to adjacent cells have been observed by Saacke and Heald.[315] They discuss the evidence that cells of a given alveolus function in synchrony regarding metabolic events; for example, an alveolus with all of its cells appearing to have fat globules of the same size and at the same stage of secretion (position in the cell) have been noted. The whole matter of intercellular communications is of profound importance. It constitutes a highly active area of research at present because of its relevance to cancer. The orientation of mammary epithelium into alveoli is the condition which differentiates them for milk synthesis and appears to suppress their replication. Continuing replication is the characteristic condition in mammary and other forms of cancer.

C. Differentiation of the mammary epithelial cell

In the area of the breasts in the young human or mammary glands of young mammals, the genetic capability exists to develop a specialized system of ducts and alveoli for the ultimate purpose of lactation. This is true of both the young male and female.

However, because of lack of adequate hormonal stimulation, the gland in the male normally will neither develop nor lactate. It can be induced to do so by a suitable program of hormone administration. In the maturing female successive heat periods or menstrual cycles release hormones that induce the development of an extensive duct system. During pregnancy the alveolar epithelium which will ultimately synthesize milk is elaborated.

It is generally held that lactation is suppressed during pregnancy by action of estrogen and progesterone of ovarian and/or placental origin on the mammary epithelium and the anterior pituitary. More specifically there appears to be an inhibitory effect of progesterone on the secretion and action of prolactin, the consummating hormone in lactation. The shedding of the placenta at parturition produces a drop in the level of progesterone and estrogen, which tends to promote lactation. Consistent with this idea is the observation that progesterone inhibits lactose synthesis by suppressing α-lactalbumin formation throughout pregnancy.[358] The removal of milk from the gland is an indispensable stimulus to its continued synthesis and secretion. There is also evidence that prostaglandin $F_{2\alpha}$ may be involved in lactogenesis.[74] We are indebted to Topper and his associates at the NIH and Cowie and coworkers in England, among others, for a considerable understanding of lactogenesis in the mammary epithelium (see reviews in refs. 179, 209 and 306). Changes are brought about in the mammary epithelial cell by a sequence of hormonal actions. The specific hormones required appear to vary somewhat from species to species, and effects may be due to hormonal interrelationships rather than exclusive actions of single hormones, but the fundamental nature of the cellular changes and that these are hormonally dependent are firmly established.

The research at Topper's laboratory with mammary tissue from mice in mid-pregnancy has produced the most detailed understanding. The first requisite is that a cell division must occur in the presence of insulin. This produces a change in the nuclear DNA which enables the daughter cell to proceed toward lactation. Without this mitosis, which involves insulin-initiated DNA synthesis, there would be no lactation, even though the subsequent events required for lactation occurred. There is some belief that insulin is simply permissive at this stage and that prolactin is the true mitogen.[249] The daughter cells resulting at this point are ultrastructurally indistinguishable from the parent cell. These cells are largely devoid of cytoplasmic membranes and organelles. The daughter cell must next be acted upon by hydrocortisone. The principal effect of this hormone is to cause a profound development of cytoplasmic membrane (rough endoplasmic reticulum) within the cell.[242] There is also some development of the Golgi apparatus at this point, but secretory vesicles are not in evidence and milk components are not yet synthesized. The essential contribution of hydrocortisone appears to be its promotion of the formation of rough endoplasmic reticulum. This membrane system is indispensable to the synthesis of the milk constituents, but with only insulin and hydrocortisone the membranes are not "turned on" to synthesize milk. Prolactin together with insulin induce the synthesis of new RNA in the nucleus and the consummating result is the synthesis of milk. The Golgi apparatus becomes hypertrophied, secretory vesicles containing casein micelles are formed in abundance and the cell takes on all of the appearances and activities of full lactation. A more detailed presentation of the nature and functioning of membranes is made later in this section.

The ultimate differentiating action of these hormones appears to lie in part with their induction of enzymes required to synthesize spermidine (see Addendum, Oka et al.). This latter compound is one which may directly influence the genome toward messengers for milk synthesis. It is generally thought that the peptide hormones act on the plasma membrane and in the case of insulin and prolactin there is some evidence to support the contention.[30,262,356] The steroid hormones are presumed to act in the nucleus. With respect to membrane synthesis it would appear that endoplasmic reticulum grows in the manner of an expanding mosaic rather uniformly over its surface. We have been unable to find any evidence of membrane subunits from the mammary cell in milk, although it contains a variety of membrane fragments and considerable cell debris.[291,348] Thus it seems unlikely that there is proliferation of membrane by accretion of subunits. The findings of Leskes et al.[215] regarding incorporation of glucose-6-phosphatase into rough endoplasmic reticulum of developing rat liver suggests its insertion all over the existing framework of the membrane system.

What happens to lactating mammary cells when they are placed in culture is somewhat conjectural at this point. There was a school of thought that such cells progressively "de-differentiate", a process in which a cell line loses its special functional capability. In the case of the mammary cell, this would involve loss of capacity to make milk components and presumably to secrete milk. A current view is that highly specialized cells, such as the lactating mammary epithelium, do not further replicate and that in culture few if any further cell divisions can be expected. Moreover, growth under culture conditions is probably not "de-differentiation" but usually the ascendency of a non-lactating cell type—frequently fibroblasts. It has been shown recently by Visser et al.[365] that a lobulo-alveolar arrangement of cells is promoted in cell cultures incubated with insulin and prolactin. There is heightened interest in culture of mammary epithelial cells as well as breast tumor cells in connection with the intensified breast cancer research program. A recent report[56] indicates that human milk is rich in viable epithelial cells. While these cells might be highly useful for metabolic studies of milk synthesis employing tracers, they may have little value as a means of growing mammary epithelium unless they can undergo transformation. For culturing of human mammary cells see Russo et al. (Addendum).

D. *Mammary lipid metabolism in relation to breast cancer*

Breast cancer is a menacing pathology of mammary epithelium. One-fourth of all deaths due to cancer among human females is caused by breast cancer. A number of kinds of mammary carcinomas require the hormone prolactin for their growth, and if prolactin is restricted these tumors will often stabilize or regress.[37] It is of interest that differentiation of mammary epithelium to lactation or to malignancy is dependent in some manner on prolactin. The principal difference is that in the one case the cell is "turned off" to replication and in the other it is "turned on". This would seem to involve the mechanism of contact inhibition at the cell surface; i.e., in the properly differentiated state the orientation of a lactating cell next to other such cells in the structure of the alveolus provides some type of input or sensitivity at the cell surface which inhibits cell multiplication. However, in the transformed or malignant state the cells are insensitive to each other's presence and proceed to replicate in an unrestricted way.

The synthesis of the glycosylating enzymes of the Golgi apparatus are under control of prolactin. It is postulated that these glycosylated lipids and proteins become recognition components of the plasma membrane, making it entirely plausible that prolactin could play a crucial role in cell surface differences. Thus prolactin seems to produce two entirely different end results from what was initially the same kind of cell. The mitogenic effect of prolactin may dominate in malignancy, whereas this characteristic is inhibited in lactation. The nature of the critical intervening events in the malignancy pathway is of course the object of intensive research.

With respect to mammals in general there seems to be no comparative data on incidence of mammary cancer. While certain experimental animals (various strains of mice and rats, the beagle dog) have proven very useful in research on mammary cancer, it is not known how susceptible they are to this malignancy compared to other species. Apparently ruminants are quite resistant to mammary cancer, but in the case of the cow diagnostic practices may be misleading. Most udder pathologies are classified as mastitis, and a chronic udder problem leads ordinarily to slaughter of the animal. Moreover, when milk production falls the animals are converted to meat so truly aged animals, the prime time for cancer, are rare. One might think that in the case of the cow numerous and prolonged lactations somehow are preventive of mammary cancer. This idea has long been prevalent with respect to breast cancer, but a recent study[226] of women from various countries has revealed that duration of lactation has no bearing on incidence of the disease. Oriental women (Japanese and Taiwanese) had relatively low incidence and American and British women higher incidence of this malignancy. Wynder[384] has postulated that fat in the diet may be a factor in breast cancer. He points to such traits as the tendency of breast cancer victims to have larger breasts, more subcutaneous fat and to be heavier than non-afflicted controls. He cites data showing that fat intake is related to the disease in humans (Fig. 7) and that this relationship is supported by a variety of animal experiments. Chan and Cohen[61] have shown that there is a greater incidence of carcin-

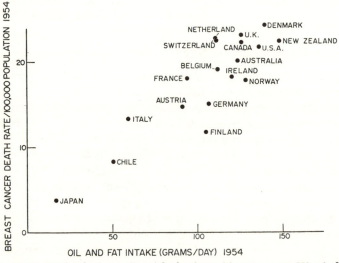

FIG. 7. Correlation between oil and fat intake and breast cancer (Wynder[384]).

ogen-induced mammary tumors in rats on a high fat diet than on a low fat diet and that tumor formation could be blocked by a prolactin-inhibiting drug.

It is notable that mammals which are quite susceptible to mammary carcinoma are monogastrics (human, dog, rat, mouse).[313] These frequently ingest considerable lipid and experience high levels of blood lipids, whereas the ruminant with its low-fat diet and multichambered stomach never seems to experience serum lipemia. We note further that lactating rat mammary tissue is usually infiltrated with adipose cells, and this condition is never normally seen in lactating cow or goat tissue. The rabbit appears to be another species that shows no fat cell infiltration of its lactating mammary epithelium and it too appears to be resistant to mammary malignancies.[313]

In the developing mammary gland new mammary epithelium extends into and tends to displace adipose tissue. The location of adipose tissue tends to define the extent of parenchymal expansion.[118] While these observations hardly establish a strong relationship between lipid metabolism and mammary cancer, they do suggest that the matter deserves research. Adipose cells could represent a reservoir for carcinogens. Such molecules might be formed, stored and/or concentrated over long periods of time in adipose cells adjacent to mammary epithelial cells. The fact that certain fat-soluble polynuclear hydrocarbons can promptly induce mammary carcinomas in rats and mice is suggestive that lipid storage might provide a crucial circumstance for the long-term formation or concentration of carcinogens. More detailed studies of food fats in the diets of women afflicted with and free of breast cancer seem needed. Comparative studies of lipid metabolism in mammary tissue of various species also should supply useful information.

E. *Lactation and the functioning of cell membranes*

For our purposes of describing and discussing metabolism in the mammary gland it is essential to consider the two remarkable and interrelated cellular processes, the synthesis and secretion of milk. A third factor bearing on the subject is maintenance of the cell; i.e., derivation of energy and continuing structural integrity.

As with all specialized cells, the lactating cell depends upon systems of membranes to accomplish its unique tasks. These membrane systems are not fundamentally different from those of other animal cells. Their structural-functional qualities are generally the same, although there are wide variations in the cellular products and tasks in which membranes of various cells participate. For the disposition of these membranes in the lactating cell see the electron photomicrograph, Fig. 8, and for a schematic presentation, Fig. 5d. Lysosomes which are few in lactating tissue are not shown. The principal cell membrane systems are as shown in the table overleaf.

Without dwelling on the many conjectural aspects of how membranes are formed and how they function we will attempt a description in light of present knowledge for the functioning of the lactating cell. Recent reviews on membranes[13,36,44,106,122,135,175,335,361] (see also *Biochimica et Biophysica Acta*, Reviews on Membranes) enable the reader to consider this subject more thoroughly. At the outset one needs to sense something of the dynamics of a highly productive cell. The cell membranes are making products and undergoing transformations simultaneously. More specifically, milk components packaged in membranes are moving through and out of the cell. Thus

Membrane	Function
Nuclear	Retention of nuclear (genetic) material, regulation of transport to and from the nucleus.
Mitochondrial	Cell respiration, oxidative phosphorylation, ATP production, metabolite synthesis and transformation.
Endoplasmic reticulum	Synthesis of lipids and proteins including enzymes, source of other cell membranes and membrane components.
Golgi	Combining and packaging of cellular products into secretory vesicles. Transformation of membranes. Glycosylation of lipids, proteins and carbohydrates.
Lysosomal	Retention and control of the release of lytic and digestive enzymes contained in lysosomes.
Plasma membrane	Retention of cell contents (defining the limits of the cell), regulation of transport into and out of the cell, recognition and communication with other cells, regulation of secretory processes and packaging of secretory products (viruses, milk fat droplets, etc.).

there is product flow and membrane flow. In order to understand this more clearly it is necessary to introduce the concepts of product vectoring and membrane flow within the cell.

1. *Vectoring of biosynthetic products within the cell*

With the exception of genetic material in the mitochondrion, the information from the nucleus for the synthesis of new products is contained in ribosomes which are either free in the cytosol (cell fluid) or bound to endoplasmic reticulum. This latter membrane exists in the form of tubes and the interior or lumen of such a tube is known as the cisterna. Thus there is an extensive interconnected plumbing system within the cell and depending on osmotic and fixative effects these cisternae may appear as collapsed layers of membranes or open tubes in electron photomicrographs of the cell. Any newly synthesized product in the cell, in consequence of these arrangements, may be vectored into the cytosol, into the membrane (endoplasmic reticulum) or into the cisternae of the endoplasmic reticulum. It seems to be consistent that secretory proteins are made on membrane-bound ribosomes and are vectored into the cisternae for transport from the cell. In fact active messenger ribonucleic acid (m–RNA) for a_s-casein (milk protein) synthesis has been detected on membrane-bound polyribosomes;[115] and until extensive rough endoplasmic reticulum (i.e., membrane with bound ribosomes) is hormonally induced in the mammary cell, no secretory protein can be synthesized. It seems likely that bound ribosomes dictate synthesis of proteins to be incorporated in the membrane, to be vectored into the cisternae of the membrane (for ultimate secretion) or to be released into the cytosol. Ribosomes free in the cytosol would be involved in synthesis of proteins to be released in the cytosol. Of course such proteins might well move to and embed in membrane surfaces. The likelihood that they would enter membrane cisternae seems somewhat more remote. In these circumstances the term enzyme can be substituted for the term protein and thus

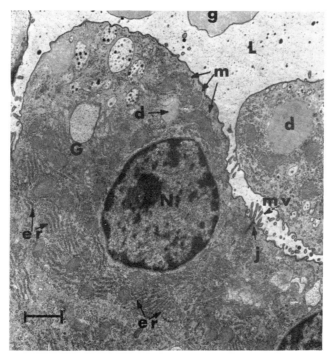

FIG. 8. An electron photomicrograph of a lactating cell (rat) with parts of several other adjoining cells. Organelles and membranes are as follows: nucleus (N) with small fat droplet (d) and mitochondria (m) above it; extensive parallel arrays of rough endoplasmic reticulum (er); Golgi vesicles (containing dark staining casein micelles) above Golgi region (G); heavily stained tight junction (j) with protruding array of microvilli (mv). Note evidence of membrane (dark line) around Golgi vesicles, limits of the cells and secreted milk fat globules (g) in lumen (L) but not around fat droplets (d) within cells. Bar (lower left) represents 1μ. (Micrograph courtesy of B. H. Stemberger).

depending on the vectoring process the proteins (enzymes) synthesized can transform the membrane surface in any one of a number of ways. They can bind to the surface of the membrane changing its synthetic or degradative capability; by enzyme action they can cause other molecules to be added to or cleaved from membrane components; and coincidental to these kinds of changes they may induce specific transport characteristics in the membranes. In summary then, the proteins synthesized on membrane-bound ribosomes and vectored into the cisternae of the membrane may not only be directed toward secretion, they also may be programmed for transforming membranes at more remote sites.

2. *Membrane transformation and flow within the cell*

The idea that an enzyme synthesized in the rough endoplasmic reticulum may be conveyed to and/or activated in some other membrane site seems to be an essential concept in accounting for cell functions. A second important consideration is that membranes like all manifestations of living systems are undergoing aging processes and various aspects of their structure are changing with time. For example, phospholipids in the cell membranes are turning over at different rates.[138,213,283] Another important factor fundamental to understanding the lactating cell concerns the constant loss of membrane in the milk secretion process. This membrane must be replaced (see section on milk secretion following).

The explanation which makes all of these properties and considerations about membranes consistent with the synthesis and secretion of milk is the idea that membranes within the lactating cell are making milk components and being transformed at the same time. New endoplasmic reticulum is being generated and this membrane in turn is passing through intermediate stages in the Golgi apparatus on the way to becoming plasma membrane. The mechanism for this transformation and flow involves the synthesis of milk constituents and their packaging for secretion in membrane-bound vesicles. A general scheme of the membrane flow-transformation concept is presented in Fig. 9. This derives from initial evidence that plasma membrane lost by the lactating cell is replaced by membranes of secretory vesicles produced in the Golgi apparatus[272,273] and from evidence that the Golgi apparatus is the site of membrane transformation from endoplasmic reticulum-like to plasma membrane-like.[121,243] Of course the fact that the endoplasmic reticulum is the membrane with primary (ribosomal) synthetic capability would suggest that in one way or another the other cell membranes are derived from it, with certain aspects of the mitochondrion excepted.[78] The unique interrelationships involved in the scheme (Fig. 9) may be better understood as the synthesis and secretion of the major milk constituents (proteins, lactose and fat) are considered.

The length of time required for ^{14}C-cholesterol to move from blood to milk in the lactating rat is 17–20 hr.[87] This seems too long a time for simple equilibration of the cholesterol throughout the plasma membrane of the lactating cell (i.e., from basal to apical regions) and is probably an indication of time required for endoplasmic reticulum to be transformed to plasma membrane.

3. *Membrane aging*

Closely related to the idea of membrane transformation and flow is the concept of membrane aging. We have noted that there is a positive correlation in the levels

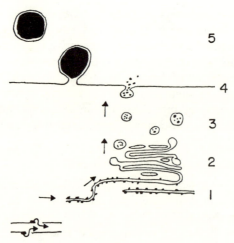

FIG. 9. A conception of the relationship between membrane flow and product flow in the synthesis and secretion of milk. Lower left: protein components of milk and enzymes involved in the synthesis of milk are vectored from ribosomes where they are made to the cisterna of the endoplasmic reticulum. The product and membrane flow in the direction of the arrows from the region of endoplasmic reticulum (1), to the Golgi apparatus, (2) where the skim milk phase is completed and packaged into secretory vesicles, (3) which fuse with and empty through the plasma membrane, (4) this membrane also accomplishes secretion of milk fat globules (dark spheres) by a packaging-type of envelopment with release into the alveolar lumen (5).

of cholesterol and sphingomyelin in membranes of the rat hepatocyte with the mitochondrion having the least and the plasma membrane the most of these two lipids.[267] The plasma membrane of bovine mammary tissue and of milk (fat globule membrane) also exhibit high levels of cholesterol and sphingomyelin (see Table 7). The question arises as to how these lipids accumulate in the plasma membrane which in a sense is asking how does the plasma membrane become what it is? An approach to these questions was afforded in experiments conducted at our laboratory to measure changes in phospholipids of plasma membrane from the lactating mammary cell.[283] ^{32}P-labeled phospholipids were produced in mammary tissue and milk by giving a lactating goat $H_3{}^{32}PO_4$ intravenously. It had been shown previously that the phosphate moiety of the phospholipids in milk are made from a pool of inorganic phosphate in mammary tissue[88] and that the phospholipids of milk exist in the form of plasma membrane around fat globules[176,272,275] and in skim milk.[291,292,348] Using these latter sources as a means of sampling plasma membrane from the cell, the radioactivity of membrane phospholipids was followed in the milk for a period of 144 hr. The data of Fig. 10 show that the specific activity of sphingomyelin progressively increased to plateau levels at about 100 hr, whereas the other phospholipids peaked and declined in specific activity. Calculation of sphingomyelin activity as a percentage of total phospholipid activity in plasma membrane from milk (Fig. 11) shows a steady increase over time. In other experiments[275] in which ^{14}C-palmitic acid was used to label the membrane phospholipids the same tendency for label to persist in the sphingomyelin was noted (Fig. 12). From these findings we interpret that sphingomyelin is more effectively retained in plasma membrane than the other phospholipids and that this characteristic is one of the factors defining how plasma membrane becomes what it is. It supports the

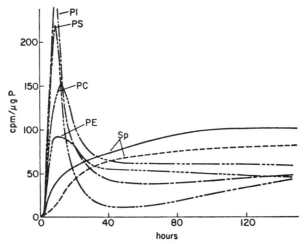

FIG. 10. Relationship between specific activity (cpm/μg P) of plasma membrane phospholipids in skim milk and the time of membrane collection (milking) following i.v. injection of $H_3{}^{32}PO_4$ into a lactating goat. — — —, Phosphatidylinositol; — – – —, Phosphatidylserine; — - - - —, Phosphatidylcholine; — - - - - —, Phosphatidylethanolamine; ———, Sphingomyelin from skim milk plasma membrane; - - -, Sphingomyelin from fat globule plasma membrane (Patton et al.[283]).

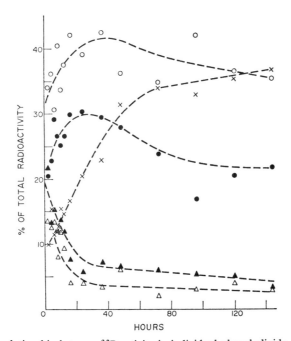

FIG. 11. The relationship between ^{32}P activity in individual phospholipids, expressed as a percentage of total ^{32}P activity in lipid of plasma membrane, and the time of membrane collection (milking) following i.v. injection of $H_3{}^{32}PO_4$ into a lactating goat. ○--○ phosphatidylcholine, ●--● phosphatidylethanolamine, ×--× sphingomyelin, ▲--▲ phosphatidylinositol and △--△ phosphatidylserine. (Derived from data of Patton et al.[283])

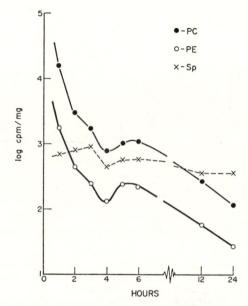

FIG. 12. The relationship between ^{14}C specific activity in individual phospholipids of plasma membrane from skim milk and the time of membrane collection (milking) following intra-mammary infusion of (^{14}C)-palmitate into a lactating goat. ● – ● phosphatidylcholine, ○ – ○ phosphatidylethanolamine and ×– –× sphingomyelin. (Data adapted from Patton and Keenan.[275])

concepts of membrane transformation and membrane aging. More particularly, given the constituents and products being made by the rough endoplasmic reticulum and the factor of time, a change of some of that membrane to other kinds of membrane (smooth endoplasmic reticulum, Golgi and plasma membrane) appears inevitable. As pointed out elsewhere, this would involve a gain in cholesterol, sphingomyelin and total lipid, a net loss in protein and certain other lipids in the case of the plasma membrane. This type of membrane aging, i.e., accumulation of cholesterol and sphingomyelin in the form of plasma membrane, has been observed in other contexts[92,213,298,312] and is related to the process of atherosclerosis.[297] For further discussion of cholesterol in relation to milk synthesis see Section IV.

4. *Synthesis of the major milk constituents*

The state of the mammary epithelial cell in which insulin and hydrocortisone have induced extensive development of rough endoplasmic reticulum yet there is essentially no evidence of milk synthesis or secretion suggests that a crucial consummating action is produced by the hormone prolactin. Prolactin appears to act at the plasma membrane[30,356] and presumably induces changes in the nucleus through a second messenger (cyclic 5' adenosine monophosphate) mechanism. The precise mode of action of prolactin at the molecular level is not yet known.

Together with insulin, prolactin induces new m-RNA and since a number of the enzymes responsible for the synthesis of milk components are known to be mediated by prolactin it is evident that the principal effect of prolactin is to cause the generation of m-RNA in the nucleus, via spermidine, which message will be translated into milk synthesis in the ribosomes of the endoplasmic reticulum.

(a) *The milk proteins.* The principal protein of most milks is the phosphoprotein, casein. Casein exists in all milks examined thus far as large micelles averaging 120 nm in diameter and with particle weights which run into the millions. In the bovine the casein micelle is comprised primarily of α-casein and lesser amounts of β- and κ-caseins. The principal unit of the casein micelle is a phosphorylated peptide of about 24,000 daltons. According to Oka and Topper,[261] casein synthesis is dependent upon sustained RNA synthesis under the influence of prolactin and in the presence of rough endoplasmic reticulum. The following sequence of events is plausible with respect to the synthesis of casein micelles. The basic peptides and the kinase(s) for their phosphorylation are synthesized on ribosomes of the rough endoplasmic reticulum.[115] These products are conveyed into the cisternae of the membrane and they flow to the Golgi apparatus where phosphorylation of the peptides occurs[29] and assembly of the casein micelle can be observed.[23] While it has been shown by Bingham et al.[29] that kinase for the phosphorylation of casein is concentrated in the Golgi apparatus, this cell structure has no protein synthetic capability and it seems most logical that the enzyme flows to that site via the lumen of the endoplasmic reticulum. Dark staining filaments, presumably phosphopeptides, can be seen (Fig. 13) in various stages of aggregation leading to casein micelle formation within the Golgi vesicle. The time required for synthesis and secretion of casein micelles in the rat or mouse mammary gland is about 30–60 min.[134,344] The origin and structure of the casein micelle has been the subject of an interpretive review by Farrell.[99] Buckheim and Welsch[55] also review this subject and present evidence that globular-shaped submicelles, 15–20 nm in diameter, are the subunits of casein micelle structure rather than filaments which are considered by them to be an artifact of fixation. Phosphate for phosphorylation of casein peptides and calcium ions for aggregation of those peptides into micelles within the Golgi appear to be derived by an ATPase.*

Other principal milk proteins include α-lactalbumin and immune globulins. β-lactoglobulin, which occurs to the extent of 0.3–0.4% in bovine milks, is known only in ruminant milks. Whether it has any cellular function and why it is primarily limited to milk of ruminants is not known. Since it is a secretory protein, its synthesis on membrane-bound ribosomes under the influence of prolactin is assumed. The regulation of α-lactalbumin synthesis by prolactin has been demonstrated[75,357] and is discussed in the following section on synthesis of lactose.

While bovine colostrum may contain as much as 16–18% of immune globulins, within a matter of days this is down to a percent or so and in several weeks it is less than 0.1%. Globulins are primarily glycoproteins and glycosylation is accomplished in endoplasmic reticulum and the Golgi apparatus. It is known that the bovine mammary cell synthesizes I_gA, I_gG, I_gM and the glycoprotein (Gpa).[57] A more extensive array of globulins is produced in human milk. Immunological properties of human milk have been reviewed by Mata and Wyatt.[231] There is a notable difference between the calf and the human infant with regard to maternal transfer of passive immunity. The calf derives most of its immune globulins by intestinal transport and very little by way of placental transport. Just the reverse is true of the human. Normally immune globulins occur on the outer surfaces of the cell and are assumed to reach this location from the Golgi apparatus by way of secretory vesicles.

---

* See Baumrucker and Keenan, Addendum.

Thus some immune globulins are disposed on the surface of milk fat globules. Immune globulins are present in the nonfat phase of milk probably by release from membrane surfaces (Golgi vesicles, cells and milk fat globules).

(b) *Lactose.* The synthesis of lactose by the lactating cell more or less outlines the entire specialized functioning of the cell. Two proteins, UDP-galactosyl transferase and α-lactalbumin, constitute the enzyme that synthesizes lactose, so-called lactose synthetase (UDP-galactose: D glucose 1-galactosyl transferase)[45,52] (see also Addendum).

$$\text{UDP galactose} + \text{glucose} \rightarrow \text{lactose} + \text{UDP}$$

Since α-lactalbumin is one of the principal (whey) proteins of milk, the synthesis of milk protein is directly related to synthesis of lactose. In the absence of α-lactalbumin glucose is not an active receptor for galactosyl transferase. In the absence of free glucose, glucosamine and bound glucose are galactosylated by the transferase. Both of the proteins of lactose synthetase are under the regulation of prolactin.[75,357] It has been shown that lactose synthetase activity is concentrated in the Golgi apparatus.[174] This provides evidence of secretory protein synthesis in the rough endoplasmic reticulum and its movement to the Golgi apparatus. However, in this case we have an example of synthesis of a product at one point on a membrane (UDP-galactosyl transferase) which leads to profound transformation of membrane properties at another point. Not only is UDP-galactosyl transferase an important enzyme in lactose synthesis, it is also considered to be the most appropriate marker enzyme for Golgi membranes from both mammary gland and liver cells.[170] Moreover, since this enzyme galactosylates a variety of glycoproteins and glycolipids which find their way to the outer surface of the cell, it is directly related to such important phenomena as cell–cell interactions, contact inhibition and immune response. No doubt enzymes of this type are the ones that make the Golgi apparatus a crucial site of membrane transformation from endoplasmic reticulum-like to plasma membrane-like. Such changes appear essential in a secretory cell, because ultimately products of this cell type must be packaged in membranes which can fuse, open and interact with other membranes and empty contents from the cell.

In summary, the knowledge of lactose synthesis now implicates cell functions extending from hormonal control of m-RNA to membrane transformation in the secretory process. Further ramifications are considered in connection with the process of secretion.

(c) *Fat.* Details of milk lipid synthesis are presented subsequently in the section dealing with biochemical pathways; we wish at this point to review aspects at the level of the cell. While lactose represents a pure chemical entity or compound and casein micelles are very large particles composed of several related species of phosphoproteins, milk fat contains a variety of triglyceride molecules. Molecular variations result from chain length, degree of unsaturation, position and geometry (*cis* or *trans*) of double bonds, chain branching, oxygenation, etc., of fatty acids as well as positioning of fatty acids on the glycerol (see Section V). Milk fat globules represent a very large accumulation of triglycerides in terms of molecular and cellular dimensions. Fat droplets within the cell and in the alveolar lumen of 8–10 μ in diameter are not uncommonly observed in cow, goat and rat mammary tissue. From electron microscopy–autoradiography studies of Stein and Stein[344] utilizing the mouse, it is evident that triglycerides are synthesized in the endoplasmic reticulum of the cell. Kinsella[188]

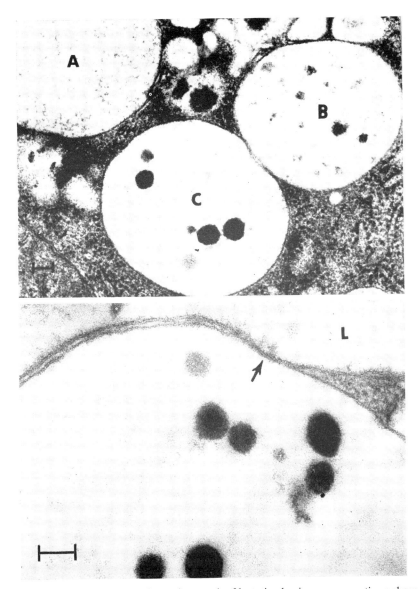

FIG. 13. Upper plate: Electron photomicrograph of lactating bovine mammary tissue showing three Golgi vesicles typical of stages in casein micelle formation: A, vesicle containing dispersion of protein filaments; B, vesicle with filaments loosely condensed; C, vesicle with filaments tightly packed into typical casein micelles as seen in milk. × 31,200. Lower plate: Portion of Golgi vesicle from lactating bovine mammary tissue. Vesicle is pressing against plasma membrane toward alveolar lumen (L). Note area where plasma membrane and Golgi vesicle membrane is fused (arrow). Dark granules within vesicle are casein micelles. × 56,800 (Beery et al.[23]).

has confirmed that milk triglycerides are recovered with the microsomal (mainly endoplasmic reticulum) fraction of the lactating cell and that this fraction is the site of milk triglyceride synthesis. However, whether it is rough, smooth or both kinds of endoplasmic reticulum that are involved was not deduced. The autoradiographic study by the Steins show the photographic grains over the rough membranes, and our own observations confirm the presence of developing fat droplets embedded in rough endoplasmic reticulum, but electron photomicrographs by Stewart[347] and by Saacke and Heald[315] show formative fat droplets in the cell may on some occasions be surrounded by arrays of smooth membranes. It is an interesting point that the ribosomes, which by their presence on the endoplasmic reticulum define it as rough, are involved in protein synthesis and so far as milk proteins and their synthesis is concerned there is good reason to believe that the key products are conveyed into the membrane cisternae. However, fat droplets appear to accumulate in a matrix of membrane and it seems reasonable that the triglyceride molecules would be synthesized and accumulated on the outer surface of the membrane rather than to be conveyed into the same tubing (leading to the Golgi apparatus) as the milk proteins and synthetase enzymes. As previously noted, a very unique difference between the liver cell and the mammary cell is that the former must direct both protein and lipid, including triglyceride, into Golgi vesicles and these are ultimately the very low density lipoproteins (VLDLs) of the blood. Essentially no lipid appears to be included in the Golgi vesicle contents of the mammary cell. This might be viewed as indicating that completely different membranes at any given time are involved in synthesizing milk proteins as opposed to milk triglycerides. This dilemma not withstanding we still must ask: How do triglyceride molecules synthesized by intracellular membranes gather into droplets?

An interesting consideration in milk fat droplet formation is the melting properties of the constituent triglycerides. Since new molecules of triglyceride must enter the growing milk fat droplet at its outer surface, a liquid state in the droplet would facilitate the uptake of additional triglyceride molecules whereas solidification of the droplet would prevent entering glyceride molecules from disappearing into the interior of the droplet. Whole bovine milk fat is completely liquid at body temperature (40°C),[333] although it contains some glycerides with much higher melting points. The ruminant mammary cell has two known devices for ensuring that milk triglycerides are maintained in a relatively liquid state. One is through synthesis of triglycerides which contain short-chain fatty acids and thus relatively low melting points. The other is through conversion of stearic acid to the lower melting oleic acid and the use of this latter acid in triglyceride synthesis. It has been shown that the *ca.* 10 mol% of butyric acid in bovine milk fat occurs 1 mole per mole of triglyceride,[83] so that *ca.* 30% of the milk triglyceride molecules contain butyric acid. Pitas *et al.*[290] and Breckenridge and Kuksis[42] have established that this butyrate is in the *sn*-3-position of the glycerol (see Table 12) so it is entirely consistent that the incorporation of this acid is a completing step in milk triglyceride synthesis.[279] Of course the other short-chain fatty acids (C_6-C_{12}) as components of triglycerides would also tend to maintain liquid conditions in milk fat droplets at body temperature. Kinsella[189] has demonstrated a close association in the stearyl desaturase and glyceride acyl transferase enzymes of lactating mammary tissue. He suggests that these two membrane-bound enzymes are physically proximate to each other on the membrane surface and that stearyl desaturase functions as a regulator of triglyceride synthesis. We are proposing that the actual cytophysical basis of this regulation may be through removal of end product (triglyceride), i.e., if the supply of oleic acid is abundant, the triglycerides will tend to be low melting and as liquid molecules can be moved easily from the site of synthesis into the fat droplet. Another consequence of this idea is that fat droplet growth may be halted by the accumulation of high melting triglycerides at its surface.

A further interesting consideration in the matter of triglyceride synthesis and milk fat droplet formation is the character and functioning of fatty acid synthetase. It appears that the unique fatty acid pattern of ruminant milk fat triglycerides is preserved so long as the mammary cells are maintained intact.[20,192] However, when fatty acid synthetase, a multienzyme complex occurring in the cytosol of the mammary cell, is isolated and purified, the exclusive product of its synthesis is palmitate.[340] This evidence suggests that within the intact cell the pattern of triglyceride fatty acids obtained may be dependent upon a structured relationship between the fatty acid synthetase and the sites of triglyceride synthesis on the endoplasmic reticulum, as appears to be the case with stearyl desaturase. We propose several possible mechanisms for milk fat droplet formation within the mammary cell. These are: (a) growth of droplets by synthesis of triglycerides at their cytoplasmic interphases (Fig. 14, upper left); (b) merging of smaller droplets to form larger droplets (Fig. 14, upper right): (c) conveyance of triglycerides by small messenger particles which are the site of triglyceride synthesis or which shuttle from that site to the forming fat droplet (Fig. 14, middle); (d) cytoplasmic flow encouraging triglyceride molecules which have accumulated by synthesis on intracellular membranes to gather into droplets in order to minimize free surface energy; formed droplet then grows in size as glyceride-laden membranes flow against it (Fig. 14, lower left); (e) conveyance of triglycerides synthesized on the endoplasmic reticulum by way of the internal non-polar phase of lipid bilayer membranes to points of glyceride accumulation (Fig. 14, lower right).

Unfortunately we do not yet have entirely adequate ways of mapping the location of lipids at the molecular level in tissues. However, some evidence in literature and our own observations with the aid of electron microscopy suggest that certain of these alternatives are less likely than others. The autoradiographic studies of Stein and Stein[344] do not indicate that the surface of forming milk fat droplets is a preferential site of glyceride synthesis, but that cell membranes (endoplasmic reticulum) are. Further, freshly secreted milk fat globules show little capability of incorporating fatty acid into triglycerides, but the skim milk phase does. So it would appear that alternative (a) is unlikely. There is no evidence as yet to support mechanisms (b) and (c). We have seldom, if ever, seen cells with many small fat droplets and we have seen very few instances of fat droplets merging, such as seems commonplace with Golgi vesicles. Rather, there are ordinarily a few fat droplets per cell. If a messenger particle of the type described in mechanism (c) exists, it has not yet been adequately demonstrated either by microscopy or biochemistry. One would expect an accumulation of such particles to be commonly observable around fat globules within the cell. Mechanisms (d) and (e) offer the alternatives that triglycerides synthesized on the membrane accumulate either on the outside or the inside of the membrane. Again we know of no consistent ultrastructural evidence to support either of these possibilities. However, if a lipid bilayer construction of the membrane at the

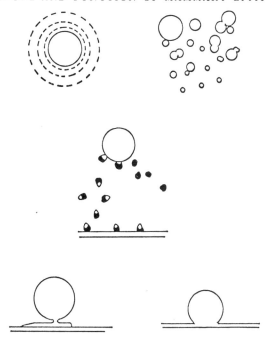

FIG. 14. Some possible mechanisms of milk fat droplet growth within cell. Upper left: droplet grows by synthesis of glycerides at its surface; upper right: droplet grows by small droplets merging to form larger droplets; middle: growth of droplet results from addition of lipid to its surface by messenger particles laden with triglyceride; lower left: droplet grows by adhesion of glycerides on surface of lipid-synthesizing membrane; lower right: droplet grows by triglycerides moving within bilayer membrane from their points of synthesis to points of accumulation (nonpolar collecting regions) (Patton [269]).

site of milk triglyceride synthesis is assumed, one might conceive of completed triglyceride molecules moving about readily within the bilayer of the membrane rather than accumulating on its more polar surface. Maintenance of a liquid condition in the hydrocarbon region of the membrane would then enable the flow of triglyceride molecules to points of accumulation (droplet formation). Skillful use of electron microscopy should eventually enable one to discern the true mechanism of milk fat droplet formation.

We have observed, as have others,[16,379] that lipid droplets in the basal area of the lactating cell are relatively small and that their mean size increases progressively toward the apical (secreting) end of the cell. Since the basal area of the cell must be relatively enriched in fatty acids of serum origin, there probably are two gradients from the basal to the apical end of the cell. One gradient involves an increase in the size of the fat droplet. The other concerns a change in the source of fatty acids for milk triglyceride synthesis. In the basal region fatty acids derived from the circulation should be an important source. Deeper within the cell and toward the secretory surface, fatty acids synthesized by the cell should be a more dominant source for triglyceride synthesis.

5. *Milk secretion*

Lipids are essential constituents of cell membranes involved in the secretion of milk. Since these membranes form structural elements of the material being secreted, milk lipids are by definition in part cell membrane lipids. Thus the ultimate end of the membrane flow process is for some of the membrane to pass into milk. There are two basic secretory mechanisms, the existence of which is supported by quite solid ultrastructural and biochemical evidence. Quite possibly other mechanisms may exist and undoubtedly our understanding of the two in question needs to be perfected in many respects, but these two do seem to account rather adequately as to how milk is secreted. One mechanism involves the flow of Golgi vesicles to the plasma membrane through which they empty their contents out of the cell into the alveolar lumen. The other mechanism concerns the enrobing of milk fat droplets with plasma membrane as they push against the limits of the cell in its apical region. This process culminates in the membrane covered fat globule being pinched off or expelled from the cell into the alveolar lumen. These two mechanisms, discussed following, appear to account for secretion of the non-fat (skim milk) and fat (globule) phases of milk respectively.

(a) *Golgi vesicle mechanism.* As suggested in the preceding section on synthesis of milk, it is a reasonable postulation that proteins to be processed by the Golgi apparatus are made by the ribosomes and associated enzymes of the rough endoplasmic reticulum and are directed into and conveyed by the cisternae of that membrane to the Golgi. These proteins involve not only those that will be secreted as such, but those that subsequently will be phosphorylated and assembled into casein micelles and enzymes for accomplishing such phosphorylation as well as those for the synthesis of lactose. These latter enzymes apparently find specific binding sites in the Golgi membranes. This raises the question of the origin of Golgi membranes (apparatus). Or to pose it another way, if the Golgi apparatus is a site of membrane transformation (endoplasmic reticulum to plasma membrane-like), what triggers the transformation? From the extensive review on origin of the Golgi apparatus by Morré et al.[243] and from the compositional studies of Golgi membrane by Keenan and his colleagues,[168,170,172] we deduce that the Golgi apparatus is not only a site of membrane tranformation, it is membrane in a state of transformation. While there may be a number of possible explanations of this basic question, we suggest that differences in turnover rates for membrane components, or in essence aging characteristics, are involved. Studies[283] of membrane labeled in the lipid phosphorus secreted into milk indicated that the various phospholipids are being incorporated and removed from the membrane at different rates (Figs. 10 and 11). The evidence suggested that the relatively high levels of sphingomyelin in plasma membrane as compared to other kinds of cell membranes is due to its relative stability or persistence in the membrane (Figs. 10–12). If endoplasmic reticulum exists primarily as an equilibrium condition, any point within it at which a molecule is removed or transformed with relative permanence represents membrane transformation. If we consider the gradient of amino acid supply to the ribosomes, it will probably be richest in the basal area of the cell, i.e., closest to the circulation, and it will become more dilute moving away from the supply toward the supranuclear region. This in fact coincides with the generally observable disposition of the rough endoplasmic reticulum. It tends to be very dense in the basal region of the cell and to give way to smooth and vesiculated membrane starting at about the nucleus and in the apical end of the cell. So transformation may coincide with diminished function (protein synthesis) of the rough endoplasmic reticulum. Of course such reactions as glycosylation of membrane proteins and lipids as occur in the Golgi apparatus will profoundly change the nature of the membranes. Two highly pertinent considerations regarding Golgi functioning from a milk secretory standpoint are osmotic effects resulting from the synthesis of lactose and the relative impermeability of plasma membrane to lactose. Linzell and Peaker[221] have proposed that an effect of lactose synthesis is to draw water into the Golgi apparatus. The conversion of glucose to lactose would lower the number of osmotically active molecules, but the actual effects would depend upon transport phenomenon involving lactose, glucose and various ions. Obviously for the making of lactose and casein micelles, glucose and calcium and phosphate ions must be supplied to the Golgi apparatus. The review of these considerations by Linzell and Peaker is instructive and should be pursued for further understanding of the plasma–cell–milk ionic relationships. Their observation that the plasma membrane of the lactating cell is impermeable to lactose strikes us as highly meaningful. This suggests that transformed membranes (plasma membrane) of the Golgi apparatus in the form of secretory vesicles actually contain lactose walled-off from the rest of the cell. One frequently hears the question why does milk contain lactose instead of glucose or some other sugar? While the question may have several correct answers it appears that the cell is removing a highly active metabolite (glucose) which might be utilized in many other pathways to a storable form (lactose isolated in Golgi vesicles).

It is now widely accepted that casein micelles are secreted from the cell by the emptying of Golgi vesicles through the plasma membrane. This was a reasonable deduction by Bargmann and Knoop[16] in their pioneering electron microscopy studies of lactating tissue and is the conclusion of ultrastructure researchers since that time, and ultrastructural evidence of the manner in which casein micelles form in Golgi vesicles can be seen in electron photomicrographs (Fig. 13). The micelles are identifiable within the vesicles in the alveolar lumen and in the milk (for example see Wellings et al.[372]) Since these micelles average 120–140 nm in diameter, it can be assumed that substantial openings through the plasma membrane need to be created so that the micelles can leave the cell. Published electron photomicrographs have purported to show this process in various stages (for example, see fig. 9b in ref. 99). While it is difficult to refute arguments that breaks in the plasma membrane in electron photomicrographs may be artifacts, casein micelles should require openings of substantial proportions to leave the cell. As discussed subsequently, the mechanism appears to involve fusion of vesicle membrane with the plasma membrane, (see Fig. 13) and emptying of the vesicle contents from the cell. It was suggested by Patton and Fowkes[272] that this might account not only for the secretion of milk proteins but lactose, the milk salts and other aqueous constituents as well, since the vesicles undoubtedly contain a suspending fluid for the casein micelles. The evidence that lactose is secreted by this mechanism is now fairly rigorous. Localization of lactose synthetase in the Golgi apparatus[174] is one point of support. The impermeability of plasma membrane to lactose[221] is also suggestive since Golgi vesicle membranes are similar to and may replenish plasma membrane. A further line of evidence is that milk protein, lactose and K^+ are all secreted at relatively the same rate[334] and this would be most unlikely for particles of such diverse size and properties unless they were emerging from the cell by the same mechanism.

The process by which Golgi vesicles merge with plasma membrane and empty their contents tends to place the inner side of their membrane in an exterior exposure at the cell surface. This is consistent with the idea that proteins and lipids glycosylated in the Golgi apparatus establish cell surface properties (immunity, contact inhibition to replication, etc.) on the exterior of the plasma membrane. It also agrees with the observation that glycoproteins are located on the cisternal interior of endomembranes.[199]

The observation that certain plant alkaloids, colchicine and vincristine, inhibit milk secretion appears to open a new area of research. The secretion process may be structured by microtubules which can be disassembled by these alkaloids (see Patton, Addendum).

(b) *Milk fat globule secretion mechanism.* For many years it was assumed that the position of materials on the surface of milk fat globules could be explained by interfacial tension relationships,[182] i.e., substances were drawn to the surface to lower tension between oil and water. However, the classic ultrastructural studies of Bargmann and Knoop[16] provided evidence that milk fat globules are secreted by extrusion into and envelopment by the plasma membrane at the apical end of the lactating cell. Many studies have since confirmed this photomicrographic observation (see Saacke and Heald[315] and Fig. 3). In addition, extensive biochemical evidence[176,272,286] has shown that the secreted milk fat globule is coated with a membrane the components of which, i.e., lipids, proteins and enzymes, are similar to those of plasma membrane. Crescents of cytoplasm are frequently occluded under the membrane around secreted globules.[381]

Both electron photomicrographs and biochemical studies indicate that lipid droplets within the cell lack such a membrane. The droplet within the cell often exhibits a thin osmiophilic line in photomicrographs which may correspond to a monolayer of lipid and protein. The surface lipid of this droplet seems to be particularly rich in phosphatidylcholine.[140,272,273] Isolation of such lipid droplets may involve artifactual gains and losses of material.

In the secretion of milk fat globules, Patton and Fowkes[272] have postulated that the lipids and proteins of the plasma membrane are attracted to the large mass of lipids of the fat droplet by London–Van der Waals' forces and hydrophobic interactions. Their calculation of the London dispersion forces indicate that an attraction force of 1 atm exists when the membrane and droplet are separated by 20Å. This force rises exponentially as the separating distance decreases.

6. *Membrane material in skim milk*

On the basis of phospholipid analysis it was suggested that the skim milk phase of bovine milk contains membrane material similar in many respects to that on the surface of secreted milk fat globules.[271] Actually analyses show that about 30–45% of the phospholipid in milk is recovered in the skim milk.[275,285] Subsequent studies[291,348] have confirmed the presence therein of vesiculated membranes and microvilli (Fig. 15). Analyses for lipid composition and enzymatic activities indicate these membrane components derive primarily from plasma membrane either directly or indirectly via milk fat globule membrane.[291,292] In particular they are rich in sphingomyelin and 5' nucleotidase. They seem to lack marker enzymes for Golgi (lactose synthetase) or endoplasmic reticulum (NADP cytochrome c reductase). However, the presence of endoplasmic reticulum is indicated by the lipogenic capabilities of these membranes.[281] Since microvilli are enriched in the membrane material of skim milk, a better opportunity to shed light on their structure and function now exists.

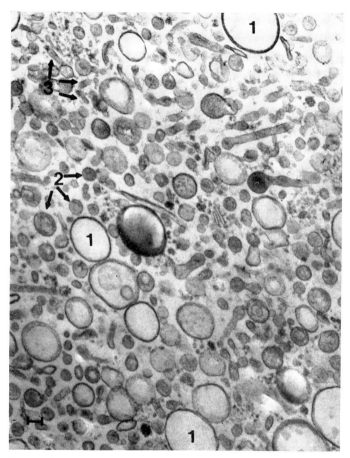

FIG. 15. The membrane or so-called fluff fraction of bovine skim milk showing at least three characteristic structures: larger vesicles the contents of which are electron transparent (1), smaller vesicles containing material that stains (2) and saclike tubes resembling microvilli (3). Bar (lower left) represents 0.1μ. (Electron photomicrograph courtesy of P. S. Stewart.)

7. *Composition of membranes from lactating tissue*

The only substantial effort thus far to reveal composition of membranes from the lactating mammary cell is that reported in a series of papers by Keenan and his colleagues.[21,22,142,143,167-170,174,176] These findings are derived from bovine tissue. It seems unlikely that profound differences in the composition of membranes from lactating tissue of most species will be encountered. We have viewed tissue from a number of species (cow, goat, rat, guinea pig, rabbit, dog). At the light and electron microscopic level there is no evidence of large species differences in the apparent structure and functioning of the alveoli. As previously noted, the cow among others is relatively devoid of interalveolar lipid deposits and thus may be more or less ideal for membrane preparation and analysis. The ready availability at the slaughter house of cows being culled from milking herds is also a facilitating factor with this species. Rabbit and guinea pig also exhibit relatively lean lactating mammary epithelium. However, the actual amount of such epithelium in the guinea pig is 55.7% of the total tissue so that one is faced with a problem of the cellular origin of membranes prepared from this tissue. On the other hand, secretory epithelium may be even more limited in other species. This problem has not yet been faced to any degree and perhaps it is not a highly significant consideration; but mammary membrane researchers should evaluate it. There are at least these kinds of tissue components that can contribute to or contaminate membrane fractions isolated from mammary tissue: endothelial cells, myoepithelial cells, leucocytes, macrophages, connective tissue, blood constituents, including red blood cells, lymph constituents and milk. Some of these components can be removed by washing and sedimentations to remove debris, but others will be entrained throughout the fractionation. A step in the right direction would involve a method for isolating mammary epithelial cells in an acceptable state of purity from the rest of the tissue.* Using these cells as starting material would enable membrane preparations to be pure with respect to cell source, but not necessarily regarding contamination of one membrane type with another from the lactating cell. The observation[56] that human milk is rich in epithelial cells provides a possible source for membrane preparations. The various kinds of cells in milk is a matter which clearly deserves research. It has been shown in our laboratories (P. S. Stewart and P. W. Todd unpublished) that several kinds of cells can be isolated from fresh milk and some of these are capable of attaching to glass when cultured *in vitro*.

(a) *Membrane preparation.* The methods used to prepare membranes from lactating mammary tissue are patterned after those developed for rat liver and are described in the previously cited papers of Keenan *et al.*[175,176] Generally the tissue is more difficult to homogenize than rat liver which disintegrates easily in a Potter–Elvehjem type homogenizer. Connective tissue occurs more abundantly in mammary tissue than in liver and this can be overcome somewhat by selective elimination when the mammary tissue is being cut into small pieces for homogenization. However, an homogenizer with moving cutting blades appears to do a superior job to a dounce-type. What one is attempting to do, of course, is to lay open as many cells as possible without producing artifactual interactions of the membranes and organelles. This is largely in the realm of an art with investigators having their various preferences. Over-homogenization tends to generate artifacts and under-homogenization makes for poor yields of membranes. The homogenate in buffer is then put through a series of

---

* In this connection, see Katz *et al.*, Addendum.

selective sedimentations and washings and resedimentations to ultimately yield membrane preparations the purity of which can be judged reasonably well by ultrastructural appearance and various compositional and marker enzyme parameters. There is a need to confirm and expand the methodology and findings of Keenan and associates on mammary tissue membranes.

(b) *Lipid composition of membranes.* The lipid composition of membrane fractions from bovine mammary tissue, as reported by Keenan and Huang, are contained in Tables 6 and 7. The lipid composition of bovine mammary mitochondria as given by those authors is presented in Table 8. Generally speaking these data, as well as those by Keenan and Morré[172] for rat liver, support the contention that Golgi apparatus is a site of membrane transformation in that its composition is in most respects intermediate between those of endoplasmic reticulum and plasma membrane. The data also demonstrate the similarity between plasma membrane and milk fat globule membrane. This is to be expected, since plasma membrane envelopes milk fat globules at secretion. The membrane material in bovine and caprine skim milk has lipid composition similar to that of bovine plasma membrane and milk fat globule membrane.[291,292] A high level of sphingomyelin (20% or more of lipid phosphorus) is characteristic of the lipids from all these sites. However, skim milk membrane does not tend to be as contaminated with triglyceride as does globule membrane. From ultrastructural appearance, lipid composition and enzymatic activity, skim milk membrane is postulated to have originated from plasma membrane.[292] However, endoplasmic reticulum might acquire such characteristics on aging in skim milk. The lipids of mitochondrial membranes, the inner membrane in particular, are rich in

TABLE 6. *Composition of Membrane Fractions from Bovine Mammary Gland* (Keenan and Huang[168])[a]

Constituent	Endoplasmic reticulum	Golgi apparatus	Plasma membrane	Globule membrane
Total lipid (mg/mg protein)	0.43 ± 0.01 (0.92)	1.24 ± 0.01 (1.36)	1.03	(1.14)
Lipid phosphorus (μg/mg lipid)	29.46 ± 1.27 (33.06)	14.27 ± 0.08 (32.2)	20.30	(31.1)
Lipid phosphorus (μg/mg protein)	12.67 ± 1.20	17.69 ± 0.13	20.91	(35.45)
Polar lipids (% of total lipids)	72.4	33.1	59.4	—
Cerebrosides (mμmoles/μg lipid P)	—	8.2	16.0	(20.0)
Cholesterol (μg/mg lipid)	36.7 ± 2.52 (54.0)	54.9 ± 9.51 (62.0)	76.0	(48.0)[b]
Ester (μeq/mg lipid)	2.34 ± .80 (2.42)	3.54 ± 0.21 (2.12)	2.20	(2.58)
Sialic acid (mμmoles/mg protein)	8.40	21.2 ± 1.03	51.0	53.5

[a]Data expressed as mean ± standard deviation of four preparations or the value obtained with four combined preparations. Figures in parentheses are values obtained with washed membrane fractions.
[b]This cholesterol content is low due to extraction of large amounts of cholesterol during the washing procedure.

TABLE 7. *Distribution of Phospholipids in Membranes from Bovine Mammary Gland* (Keenan and Huang[168])[a]

	Percent of total lipid phosphorus			
Phospholipid	Endoplasmic reticulum	Golgi apparatus	Plasma membrane	Globule membrane
Sphingomyelin	5.7 ± 0.26 (5.2)	12.7 ± 1.68 (11.7)	19.6	19.1(19.1)
Phosphatidyl choline	57.1 ± 3.99 (55.1)	46.8 ± 1.82 (46.4)	38.9	38.0(34.8)
Phosphatidyl serine	4.1 ± 0.98 (3.9)	6.0 ± 1.02 (5.0)	6.4	5.0 (5.0)
Phosphatidyl inositol	5.7 ± 1.39 (6.6)	7.1 ± 1.91 (8.1)	5.8	8.0 (9.0)
Phosphatidyl ethanolamine	23.6 ± 1.59 (27.2)	27.1 ± 2.99 (24.9)	24.1	27.4 (29.4)
Lysophosphatidyl choline	1.6 ± 0.39 (0.8)	0.4 ± 0.31 (2.8)	3.4	1.7 (2.3)
Lysophosphatidyl ethanolamine	2.1 ± 1.50 (1.3)	0.1 ± 0.22 (1.0)	0.9	0.6 (0.3)
Cardiolipin	0.2 ± 0.40	—	0.8	—

[a]Results expressed as mean ± standard deviation of four separate preparations or as the value obtained with four combined preparations. Figures in parentheses are values obtained with washed membrane fractions.

TABLE 8. *Lipid Distribution in Bovine Mammary Mitochondria* (Huang and Keenan[142])[ab]

	Percent of	
Lipid component	Total lipid	Total lipid phosphorus
Total phospholipid	84.7 ± 1.06	
Lysophosphatidyl choline		0.88 ± 0.02
Lysophosphatidyl ethanolamine		1.17 ± 0.60
Sphingomyelin		3.03 ± 0.58
Phosphatidyl choline		43.18 ± 1.20
Phosphatidyl serine		0.36 ± 0.07
Phosphatidyl inositol		4.89 ± 0.28
Phosphatidyl ethanolamine		25.06 ± 0.55
Cardiolipin		17.84 ± 0.65
Unidentified phospholipids[c]		3.59 ± 0.18
Total neutral lipid	15.3 ± 1.10	
Cholesterol	3.34 ± 0.16	
Free fatty acids	6.67 ± 0.42	
Triglycerides	2.04 ± 0.11	
Diglycerides	1.14 ± 0.14	
Cholesterol esters + hydrocarbons	2.07 ± 0.29	

[a]Lipid to protein ratio, mean value 0.35.
[b]Values are means plus and minus standard experimental errors, $n = 4$.
[c]Composed of a total of three unidentified components.

cardiolipin. This is shown by the data of Huang and Keenan[142] who found that about 18% of the phospholipids of bovine mammary mitochondria are accounted by this lipid. This is somewhat higher than the values reported earlier by Patton et al.[274] of 10–14% cardiolipin in phospholipids of mitochondria from bovine and caprine mammary tissue.

(c) *Protein composition of membranes.* The data on protein composition of membranes from bovine mammary tissue are very limited. Beyond the analyses of Keenan and Huang[168] the findings are limited to the milk fat globule membrane. The polyacrylamide gel electrophoretic separation of proteins from rough endoplasmic reticulum, Golgi apparatus and milk fat globule membrane of bovine mammary tissue reveals a complex pattern of some 25 components.[168] Eight of these were present in all three types of membrane. A previous study[176] showed a very similar pattern of proteins in the plasma membrane and the milk fat globule membrane. Early studies established that the bovine milk fat globule membrane is rich in glycoproteins.[54] Recent studies,[196,229,255] using the powerful resolution capable with gel electrophoresis, have shown that there are at least five or six different glycoproteins in both bovine and human milk fat globules. Some of these are sialoglycoproteins on the outer surface of the globule. Newman and Harrison[255] conclude from their findings on glycoproteins in the outer surface of the bovine milk fat globule that it must have derived from the plasmalemma (plasma membrane) of the alveolar cell.

F. *Critique of observations of secretory phenomena*

There has been a strong surge of interest in the physiology and biochemistry of the lactating mammary cell during the past 15 years. This cell offers certain advantages as an object of study. Under hormonal influence it differentiates rather dramatically, it is very active metabolically; because of its synthetic and secretory activity, it is involved in diverse membrane phenomena; and its product, milk, provides a record of cell activity. The problem of breast cancer is an additional motivating factor for study.

Application of the electron microscope has been indispensable to progress in understanding the structure and function of the lactating cell. However, many of the controversial points in this understanding have arisen over interpretation of data provided by this tool. On the other hand, the biochemical approach has limitations at the various levels that it has been applied (homogenate, cell culture, tissue slice, etc.) and it is evident that the two approaches should be used to reinforce each other so far as possible. Due to limitations in amounts and quality of data being produced by these approaches a number of healthy controversies exist regarding secretory mechanisms and milk fat globule membrane structure and properties. The issues are central to an understanding of membranes. Moreover, their discussion may highlight the need for certain kinds of research.

1. *Golgi secretory process*

It has been proposed by Patton and Fowkes[272] that plasma membrane removed from the cell incident to secretion of milk fat globules is replenished by merging of Golgi vesicle membranes with the plasma membrane at the time these vesicles empty their contents from the cell. While this seems plausible, the problem of what maintains balance in the situation needs to be examined. If the Golgi vesicles contain what is essentially the nonfat phase of milk (skim milk), then they are accounting for secretion of over 90% of the milk volume in most species. The milk fat globules which are relatively tightly packaged in membrane are composed almost exclusively of lipid which represent 3–6% of bovine milk volume. So the ratio of milk volume secreted by Golgi vesicles may be some 20 times that for milk fat globules. Even if a substantial amount of the water in milk is derived by other transport than Golgi vesicles, this ratio may still favor larger milk volume moving via vesicles. Actually we find from counting casein micelles in mature Golgi vesicles on photomicrographs that numbers of casein micelles per unit area in mature Golgi vesicles are of the same order of magnitude as those for alveolar lumen; so there does not appear to be a large dilution of vesicle content in its transfer to milk.

In addition, Golgi vesicles are considerably smaller on an average than fat globules. Thus it would appear, considering their greater number, their greater volume and their smaller size, that they involve far more membrane surface than would be needed to replenish the plasma membrane loss from the cell by milk fat globule secretion. One possible explanation may be that excess plasma membrane is resorbed, although no evidence of this has been presented. Another explanation is that the Golgi vesicle membrane system may be a more stable framework within the cell than is apparent from micrographs. It looks to be a collection of bubbles that are growing and flowing. Possibly it may function more in the manner of a flexible lattice through which the milk fluid percolates. In this case the movement of membrane to the plasma membrane would be quite limited. It is of interest in this connection that drugs which inhibit microtubule function (colchicine and vinblastine) prevent secretion of serum lipoproteins from Golgi vesicles in the liver.[263,345] This may be a problem in Golgi vesicle interaction or fusion with the plasma membrane. Recent evidence[383] indicates that colchicine interferes with the mobility of plasma membrane particles. Orci et al.[263] and Stein and Stein[345] suggest that colchicine inhibits the Golgi vesicle transport by interacting with microtubules.

2. *Fat globule secretion*

We have noted that the process by which the milk fat droplet forms within the cell is not known (p. 203). Nor is it known what forces move the droplet to the apical region of the cell or how long this process may take. From numerous fatty acid labeling experiments we estimate that the average milk fat globule is synthesized in a period of 4–6 hr in the goat.

The proposal[272] that London–Van der Waals' forces attract the plasma membrane to the surface of the milk fat droplet in the secretion process has been criticized in ultrastructure studies by Wooding.[379] He has measured the distance between what appears to be plasma membrane and fat droplet surface in electron photomicrographs of secreted globules and finds an intervening zone too large in diameter (10–20 nm) to justify the invocation of London–Van der Waals' forces for such an attraction. Both the distance over which such forces may be effective and the distance between the membrane and the droplet surface in the living animal are somewhat conjectural. It does seem true that there are strong attraction forces in that secreted milk fat globules are not just loosely occluded in membrane. The majority of globules appear to be quite smoothly, and to some extent inextricably,[177] encased over most of their surface. No doubt other hydrophobic interactions in addition to London–Van der Waals' forces are involved in the attraction between the membrane and the fat droplet. On the other hand, it may be risky to assume that distances between cell structures are preserved with infinite accuracy by the procedures used for electron microscopy. For example, it has been shown that the red cell membrane varies in diameter and appearance depending on the fixation procedure.[305] One also wonders what kinds of changes in spatial relationships at the nanometer level take place when milk or tissue are cooled from body temperature to room temperature or refrigerating temperature. Interestingly enough this kind of treatment is used to dissociate the subunits of fatty acid synthetase[340] and in the case of freezing and thawing to dissociate membrane from the surface of milk fat globules.[5,86,275]

3. *Fat globule membrane**

In this connection one of the most significant controversies concerns what if any membrane resides on the surface of secreted milk fat globules. We have contended that the milk fat globule is a remarkable model for the study of membrane phenomenon because (1) it isolates (in milk) plasma membrane from the cell in a physiological manner that does not require homogenizing and fractionating tissue with the artifacts attendant such treatment; (2) the secretion mechanism occludes the inner surface of the plasma membrane and exposes the outer surface thus enabling an approach to sidedness of the plasma membrane; (3) the fact that milk fat globules can be obtained from virtually any mammalian species facilitates membrane comparisons. While it is generally conceded by a number of microscopists that there is some change apparent in the milk fat globule membrane following secretion,[15,18,136,347,378] it is not clear what the character or degree of this change is and how rapidly it occurs.

The general consensus of electron microscopists is that no unit membrane surrounds the fat droplet within the cell, that such a membrane envelopes the droplet at secretion, that there is a change in the appearance of the membrane on the globule post-secretion, but that it is still evident that the secreted globule is enveloped in a much more electron dense layer than intracellular droplets. Wooding concludes from ultrastructural studies[378-380] that most of the initial milk fat globule membrane is lost into the milk plasma by a process of vesiculation, leaving a structureless secondary milk fat globule membrane as the only continuous boundary to the milk fat globule. Of course if this is true the milk fat globule membrane would have somewhat restricted value for purposes of membrane or cellular research. In his ultrastuctural studies Bauer[18] claims that some loss of membrane from milk fat globules is produced by their preparation (fixation) for electron microscopy. Keenan *et al.*[177] have shown that membranes of milk fat globules have reasonably good unit membrane appearance, although they tend to bind glyceride material on their inner surface.

Is it not possible that the post-secretion change in the appearance of the milk fat globule membrane is due somewhat to a continuation of dehydration effects initiated by the forces attracting the membrane onto the fat droplet in the first place? It seems reasonable that hydrophobic forces of this type would continue to act after secretion, expelling additional water (cytoplasm) and pulling the membrane more and more tightly onto the globule. Bearing in mind the difficulties of lipid fixation, we feel that differences in appearance of membrane around aged globules may result from progressing dehydration of the membrane which makes it more difficult to fix, embed and section. Wherever globules contain cytoplasmic inclusions (moisture) under the membrane, definition of the membrane under the electron microscope is improved (fig. 10, ref. 136).

In analyzing the problem of fat globule membrane stability, it seems desirable to review events and observations from the standpoints of both cytology and biochem-

---

* For further recent literature, see Addendum.

istry. At the outset the time factor needs to be considered. Biochemists would admit that a membrane preparation has some finite life regarding its usefulness for research. The manner in which milk or tissue is recovered and what is done with it until observations are made clearly represent significant variables. Cows are normally milked twice a day and they deliver milk from their udders which is on average quite a few hours post-secretion from cells. Some small fraction of the milk in their gland at any time is at least 24 hr old. Because milk will keep well microbiologically when refrigerated at 2–4°C, it is now accumulated in bulk tanks for several days before delivery to U.S. plants. Such cold, old, raw milk probably has limited value for membrane studies. The mere volume of milk that is held up in the completely milked bovine gland represents a problem in the objective of obtaining freshly secreted milk. For many experimental purposes we use a goat when the object is to obtain freshly secreted milk. The goat is completely milked and then milked for 2 or 3 hr at ½-hr intervals. Under these conditions most of the residual milk will have been removed.

As previously stated, three principal surfaces are involved in the freshly secreted milk fat globule. There is the native surface that it had as a fat droplet before secretion from the cell, and there are the inner and outer surfaces of the plasma membrane which are super-imposed on the native surface (Fig. 2). While it is well known that the core of the milk fat globule is composed almost exclusively of glycerides, the native surface probably represents unique pools of cholesterol, phospholipids, proteins and other surface-active molecules. Thus whether one is analyzing enzyme activities, cholesterol or phospholipid, etc., it is not possible to assume that globule surface material is entirely plasma membrane. Material within cytoplasmic crescents poses a further consideration (see following).

Most of the lipid phosphorus and cholesterol in milk is associated with the milk fat globules. Milks (cow and goat) normally collected from the gland have ca. 60% of their phospholipid and ca. 85% of their cholesterol associated with milk fat globules. The phospholipid distribution and activity of certain enzymes (5' nucleotidase and ATPase) of the milk fat globule have been shown to be stable in cows milk for at least 96 hr.[21] These data indicate that in fresh milk there is very little shedding of membrane material from the globule surface into the skim milk. However, as noted previously, milk is to some extent 'old' at milking and material could be lost from milk fat globules immediately following their release from the cell. Plasma membrane of the cell might be especially susceptible to vesiculation as it reassembles behind expelled milk fat globules. It may prove difficult to establish whether membrane material in skim milk comes from plasma membrane of the cell directly or by way of the milk fat globule membrane.

Another line of evidence, presented by Kobylka and Carraway,[197] purports to show that the milk fat globule membrane is in a disintegrated state because of the relative digestibility of the membrane proteins by tryptic-type enzymes. Their basis of comparison was the red blood cell membrane. The main purpose of the red cell membrane is to regulate transport of small molecules and ions. The principal purpose of the plasma membrane of the lactating mammary cell is to secrete large particles of protein and fat, and this membrane is laden with many different proteins derived from its synthetic and secretory roles. In addition, it may be turning over much more rapidly and have structure and function quite at variance with that of the red blood cell or of many other kinds of cells for that matter. The digestibility of membrane proteins by enzymes, even of red blood cells, appears to be a relative matter.[44] In cell culture preparation it is well known that prolonged treatment with tryptic-type enzymes will disintegrate most cells. While the membrane of the milk fat globule may indeed be somewhat disintegrated depending on its age, we would expect it to have some properties at variance with the membrane of the red blood cell.

There is evidence to suggest that shedding of milk fat globule membrane cannot fully explain the origin of the membrane material in skim milk. A significant portion of the latter has ultrastructural characteristics of microvilli[348] and these more likely arise from cell surfaces than milk fat globules. A lack of Mg^{2+}-activated ATPase in skim milk membrane has been noted,[291] in contrast to substantial activity characteristic of fat globule membrane preparations.[86,230,286] *In vivo* labeling experiments[275] with ^{14}C-palmitate have evidenced much more extensive incorporation of activity into skim milk membrane than into milk fat globule membrane. We also suspect that there is much less carotene associated with bovine skim milk membrane than with milk fat globule membrane of that species, although this has not yet been precisely measured.

Considering the variety of cell types in mammary tissue and milk and the amount of cellular debris entering milk, multiple origins of the skim milk membrane material seems likely. At least three types of material can be discerned (Fig. 15): vesicles the contents of which are electron transparent, smaller vesicles containing material that is stained to varying degrees and sloughed microvilli. In any event, understanding of the origin and nature of this material will benefit from further research. Recent evidence indicates that it has some of the properties of plasma membrane[292] and that the levels of it vary with milking practice.[285]

4. Globule crescents

A further issue about structure of milk fat globules and the mechanism of their secretion concerns the occurrence of so-called crescents of cytoplasm. Wooding et al.[381] have noted that 1–5% of bovine milk fat globules include crescents containing cytoplasm with or without endoplasmic reticulum, mitochondria, etc. On the basis of the extremely small volume of milk involved, we[268] questioned the significance of this as the basis of defining milk secretion as apocrine, Linzell[219] presented a magnificent defense of the importance of small things; so there is no question about the observable in this issue, it is a matter of semantics. On the basis of the amount of cardiolipin in milk and mammary tissue (observed ratio, one to several hundred) as a marker for mitochondria, Patton et al.[274] have shown that the loss of cytoplasmic material from the lactating cell must be very limited. Their data imply that secretion occurs with little or no loss of cell integrity.

5. Sidedness of plasma membrane

As previously mentioned, the milk fat globule provides an approach to the sidedness of plasma membrane, since the secretion mechanism exposes the outer surface of this membrane on the milk fat globule. In an investigation of this approach, Patton and Trams[286] assayed the specific activity of several enzymes on intact globules and on membrane material released from globules by churning. The specific activities of the enzymes (nmoles/min/mg protein) in the two positions respectively were: 5' nucleotidase 192 and 205, nucleotide pyrophosphate 42 and 159, Mg^{2+}-activated ATPase

10.7 and 15. From these data it was reasoned that the 5' nucleotidase was in the outer surface, since releasing the membrane from the globule and refining it produced little change in specific activity. Variations in activity for the other two enzymes suggest that they may at least partly occur on the inner membrane surface. Kobylka and Carraway[197] have cautioned that this type of experimental assumption may be erroneous on the basis of their findings and those of Wooding[378] that the milk fat globule membrane is a disintegrated plasma membrane. More recently Martel et al.[229] have concluded that the milk fat globule membrane is a mixture of membranes because it contains marker enzymes for endoplasmic reticulum, Golgi apparatus and plasma membrane. Actually such enzymes are found in bovine milk fat globule membrane also.[86,286] We feel that such observations are consistent with the concept of membrane transformation expounded previously. We postulate that the milk fat globule membrane evolved from rough endoplasmic reticulum, to Golgi apparatus membrane, to Golgi vesicle membrane, to plasma membrane and on to milk fat globules. In a secretory cell this membrane evolution may happen rather rapidly because of membrane turnover into milk. It may well produce a secretory membrane with some remaining characteristics of the endomembranes of the cell and with special features to facilitate secretion.

We find it interesting that the isolation of 5' nucleotidase from plasma membrane has witnessed parallel enrichment of enzyme activity and sphingomyelin.[144,375] While sphingomyelin apparently is not an essential component of the enzyme,[97] other lines of evidence indicate that it is on the outer surface of the plasma membrane.[44] Thus the enrichment of 5' nucleotidase and sphingomyelin is consistent with their existing in proximity to one another in the outer surface of the plasma membrane.

It is perhaps worth stressing that mere demonstration of a so-called marker enzyme in a membrane does not necessarily imply either homogeneity or contamination of that membrane material. As pointed out by Solyom and Trams, isozymes may be involved with different forms of the enzyme being associated with different membranes (see their excellent review[342] for discussion of 5' nucleotidase in liver cell membranes). Moreover, it appears that the Golgi apparatus, for example, has no protein synthesis capability (little or no nucleic acid), so that its marker enzyme, UDP galactosyl transferase, is at least in part made elsewhere and may be found to some extent in the endoplasmic reticulum. Comparative specific activity rather than mere presence of an enzyme would seem to give guidance on significance of marker enzyme findings.

IV. BIOCHEMICAL PATHWAYS IN TISSUE AND MILK LIPID SYNTHESIS

A. *Introduction*

Regarding this section dealing with metabolic pathways and the following section on composition of milk lipids, it is well to remember that milk is not just a collection of various kinds of molecules. Its lipids are best understood as a biological display of products put out by a cell. They are found in membranes and products wrapped in membranes. The milk fat globule as previously described should be considered in terms of compartments such as its triglyceride core, the surface it had within the cell and the (membrane) material that was added to it at secretion. Even though we have no completely acceptable way as yet to isolate these compartments for study, it is helpful to conceptualize the lipids this way. For example, in thinking about the cholesterol and phospholipids of milk, it is reasonable to suspect that the surface of the milk fat droplet in the cell prior to secretion contains some of these lipids. This appears to be the case.[140] And if cholesterol is present therein in free and esterified form it would be plausible to assume that the esterified cholesterol might be dissolved in the glyceride core and the free sterol disposed at the droplet surface as is indicated for these components in serum lipoproteins (see p. 68). Additional pools of phospholipid and free and esterified cholesterol would be expected to exist in the plasma membrane around the fat globule and in the membrane material of skim milk. In light of evidence that 5' nucleotidase is on the outer surface of the milk fat globule (and plasma) membrane[286] and that it is isolated with lipids containing a high concentration of sphingomyelin[144,375] one can suppose that sphingomyelin also is in the outer surface of the membrane. In the use of NH_2-group binding agents in their study of milk fat globule membrane, Newman and Harrison[255] do not indicate the isolation of products from phosphatidylethanolamine or phosphatidylserine among the NH_2-derivatives isolated, which suggests that these phospholipids are on inner membrane surfaces of the fat globule and the cell plasma membrane. These lines of evidence for placement of membrane lipids are consistent with those reviewed for other cell types by Bretscher.[44] Ultimately, we would like to know where each type of molecule is in the milk fat globule, and sidedness of its surface membrane affords an opportunity to expand understanding of cell membranes (see also review by Patton and Keenan, Addendum).

The metabolism of lipids in mammary tissue falls into three general categories: synthesis for incorporation into cellular structures, particularly membranes; synthesis for secretion into milk; and catabolism for energy purposes. Actually so far as the lactating mammary cell is concerned the synthesis of its structural lipid substantially overlaps the matter of milk lipid synthesis because, as discussed in the previous section, the membranes of the cell evolve into the milk as a result of secretory mechanisms. Thus the synthesis of the phospholipids, glycolipids, cholesterol, etc., of milk are actually manifestations of structural lipids in the cell. On the other hand, the triglycerides of milk which constitute better than 95% of the total milk lipids can be treated much more clearly as a product of the cell rather than an indispensable aspect of its structure.

By way of review, Fig. 4 outlines the metabolites in the blood that are taken up by the mammary gland. These are principally: amino acids, glucose, acetate, β-hydroxybutyrate, triglycerides (in chylomicrons and VLDLs), free fatty acids and cholesterol. In addition, various ions and trace amounts of many other serum components are transported into milk. The amino acids are utilized primarily for protein synthesis. A number of the other substrates are utilized both for synthesis of lipids and for energy purposes as discussed following.

B. *Energy metabolism of mammary tissue*

While the precise respiratory activity of lactating mammary epithelial cells is not yet defined, even for a particular species, physiologists have revealed a number of interesting facts about mammary tissue from tracer studies with perfused glands as well as with intact animals. Although the tissue is a complex of cell types, the findings necessarily implicate the lactating cell. Moreover, it is reasonable to assume, as with most actively respiring mammalian tissues, that the mitochondrion in the mammary cell generates ATP for energy requiring reactions and cell functions from such metabolites as fatty acids, glucose, etc. Some of the most definitive and extensive studies of the matter are those of Annison, Linzell and their associates[7,8,220,221] using the lactating goat. One of the more interesting observations from their studies is that long-chain fatty acids from the blood are a very minor source of CO_2 production by lactating mammary tissue. They find that about two-thirds of mammary CO_2 derives from acetate and glucose with propionate and butyrate as probable additional sources. They report further that 60–85% of the total glucose produced in the body is utilized by the lactating goat mammary gland. This is a tremendous increase from minor utilization of the metabolite by the dry gland. Glucose provides substrate for lactose synthesis, glycerol for lipid synthesis and 29–49% of mammary CO_2. Of course the ruminant is unique for its generation of acetate (in the rumen) as a key body metabolite. According to Annison and Linzell,[7] 15–41% of the acetate in a lactating goat is used by the mammary gland and of this 29–69% is oxidized, the rest being used mainly for fatty acid synthesis, in particular for the short- and medium-chain length acids (C_4–C_{16}) which are incorporated into milk fat triglycerides. It is frequently stated that approximately 50% of the acetate taken up by the ruminant mammary gland is oxidized and about 50% is used for milk fatty acid synthesis.

There appear to be no data for respiratory metabolism of lactating tissue in non-ruminant species. Acetate would be somewhat less important and glucose and fatty acid more important in the human and other monogastrics. In addition, it is well established that glucose is a source of acetate for fatty acid synthesis in the non-ruminant mammary glands. There are significant differences in the metabolic pathways of glucose and acetate in ruminants and non-ruminants (see Ballard et al.[12]).

The synthesis of fat in mammary epithelium involves conversion of acetate in the cytoplasm and probably in the mitochondrion to the main substrate for fatty acid synthesis, acetyl-CoA. To support lipogenesis a sufficient supply of NADPH for hydrogenation is required. As shown by Ballard et al.,[12] the enzyme systems in the mitochondrion and in the cytoplasm of rat mammary tissue are adequate to generate these essentials from glucose, whereas in the ruminant the lack of citrate cleaving enzyme depresses the yield of acetate and oxalacetate from glucose. The oxalacetate is required for synthesis of an adequate supply of NADPH. However, we have noted in experiments (S. Patton and R. D. McCarthy; G. D. Coccodrilli and R. D. McCarthy, unpublished) involving intramammary infusion of ^{14}C-glucose into the lactating goat that some 10–20% of the label incorporated into the triglycerides was found in the fatty acids, the remainder being in the glycerol. There may be individual animal variations and stress situations that enable a significant utilization of glucose for milk fatty acid synthesis even in the ruminant.

C. Fatty acid synthesis

The principal purpose of fatty acid synthesis in mammary tissue is to provide acyl groups for the production of triglycerides for milk fat globules. In the ruminant, mammary gland acetate and β-hydroxybutyrate derived from the circulation are the two important substrates for fatty acid synthesis. In the non-ruminant, these metabolites from the blood are strongly supplemented by acetate derived in the mammary cell from glucose. This latter pathway involves conversion of glucose to triose phosphate via the Embden–Meyerhof pathway, conversion of triose phosphate to pyruvate, formation of citrate from pyruvate in the tricarboxylic acid cycle of the mitochondrion and cleavage of citrate diffusing from the mitochondrion to acetate and oxolacetate. The conversion of oxolacetate to pyruvate and the metabolism of glucose through the pentose phosphate cycle yield the necessary NADPH for reduction of the acetyl groups in their condensation to form the fatty acids. An excellent presentation of the schemes and mechanisms of these classic pathways in relation to the synthesis of milk fatty acids is given by Bauman and Davis.[19,70]

1. Enzymes

There are two principal enzyme complexes involved in fatty acid synthesis by mammary tissue: acetyl CoA carboxylase and fatty acid synthetase.[227,367] The former enzyme appears to be composed of at least three functional protein components one of which contains biotin. This enzyme accomplishes the conversion of acetyl CoA to malonyl CoA, an essential reactant in the malonyl CoA pathway. The reaction requires ATP and is an interesting example of CO_2 fixation by animal tissue. The precise cellular location of acetyl CoA carboxylase is uncertain. Sub-cellular fractionations find it disposed (loosely bound) in the microsomal pellet and in the supernatant with some species variations.

Fatty acid synthetase is a multi-enzyme complex of about 500,000 mol. wt. located in the cytoplasm of the cell. Characterizations of the complex from mammary tissue and liver of a number of species indicate it to be quite similar in its properties from these various sites.[19] In fact the evidence of Smith[339] is quite convincing that fatty acid synthetases of rat liver and mammary gland are essentially identical. A crucial component of the complex is acyl carrier protein (ACP) containing a 4-phosphopantetheine group. This protein serves as the vehicle for reactants in a series of enzymatic condensations and reductive conversions. In essence, acetyl CoA and malonyl CoA are converted to the ACP derivatives and condensed to acetoacetyl ACP. This latter intermediate is reduced via β-hydroxybutyryl and crotonyl derivatives to butyryl ACP. Lengthening of the fatty acid chain by successive two carbon units is accomplished through additions of malonyl ACP to the carboxyl end of the chain. The net reaction in the formation of palmitate by fatty acid synthetase is:

$$\text{Acetyl CoA} + 7 \text{ Malonyl CoA} + 14 \text{ NADPH} \rightarrow \text{Palmitate} + 7 CO_2 + 14 \text{ NADP} + 8 \text{ CoA}$$

A further group of enzymes appears to be involved in a mechanism which synthesizes butyryl CoA from acetyl CoA in mammary tissue by reversal of β-oxidation[218] (see following on sources of carbon and pathways).

As pointed out by Smith and Abraham,[340] a particularly interesting feature in studying fatty acid synthetase derives from its being, rather than one enzyme, a naturally organized conglomerate of enzymes required to accomplish an interrelated sequence of reactions. They find that the complex is held in a functional state by hydrophobic interactions that can be suppressed by cooling. Further information on composition and properties of acetyl CoA carboxylase, fatty acid synthetase and acyl carrier protein is available in reviews.[19,227,359,367]

Another enzyme of crucial importance in fatty acid metabolism of ruminant mammary tissue is stearyl desaturase.[8,189,210] This enzyme, which converts stearic acid to oleic acid, is associated with the microsomal fraction of the tissue and in all likelihood it is concentrated in the endoplasmic reticulum of the lactating cell. The reaction utilizes stearyl CoA as substrate and is facilitated by NADH.[189] It acts in fresh goat's milk simply on addition of stearic acid.[236]

While the enzyme is relatively specific for stearic acid, it appears probable that other milk fatty acids are desaturated at a much slower rate. The series of even carbon numbered *cis* 9-enoic acids of milk fat, C_{10} through C_{16} (see Section V), in addition to oleic, presumably originate by stearyl desaturase action in mammary tissue.

Bauman and Davis[19] indicate that some non-ruminant mammary tissues (rat and rabbit) lack the enzyme, while that of the pig contains it. Considering the fact that ruminant digestive metabolism makes mainly stearic and palmitic acids available in the organism, it is readily evident why ruminant tissues might require stearyl desaturase. Fluidity of membranes and of lipid droplets would require a certain degree of unsaturation.

Except for enzymes involved in synthesis of the amide-linked fatty acids of the sphingolipids, which are rich in C_{22}, C_{23}, and C_{24} carbon chain lengths, there appears to be very little chain elongation activity in mammary tissue. This is evident from the many studies utilizing acetate in which little or no labeling was observed in the C_{18} milk fatty acids, e.g. Popjak *et al.*,[296] Lawrence and Hawke,[212] and Walker *et al.*[368]

2. *Sources of carbon and pathways*

At our laboratory the administration of acetate-C^{14} to the lactating goat yielded reproducible labeling of the C_{10}, C_{12}, C_{14} and C_{16} fatty acids of the milk fat.[368] There was considerably less labeling of the C_4, C_6, and C_8 or C_{18} acids under these conditions and all of these acids are significant components of goat milk fat. It seems certain that the fatty acids labeled in this experiment were being synthesized primarily by the malonyl CoA pathway. It is known that there is a non-malonyl (avidin insensitive) pathway of fatty acid synthesis in mammary tissue for the C_4 fatty acid[205] and the C_6 and C_8 fatty acids as well.[239] This has led Dimick *et al.*[82] to suggest three principal

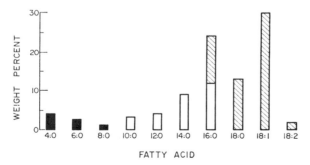

FIG. 16. Characteristic fatty acid composition of ruminant milk lipids showing probable sources of the fatty acids: ■ non-malonyl-CoA pathway in mammary tissue, □ malonyl CoA pathway in the tissue and ▨ from circulating blood lipids (Dimick *et al.*[82]).

sources of fatty acids for synthesis of ruminant milk fat as shown in Fig. 16. These are the C_4, C_6 and C_8 fatty acids synthesized primarily by an avidin insensitive pathway involving β-hydroxybutyrate as substrate; the C_{10} through C_{14} and part of the C_{16} fatty acids synthesized by the malonyl CoA pathway; and the remaining C_{16} and all of the C_{18} fatty acids being derived from the circulation.

Lin and Kumar[218] have supplied evidence that butyryl CoA is synthesized from acetyl CoA by reversal of β-oxidation in mammary tissue. They have shown further that in rat mammary gland and liver, but not in adipose tissue, butyryl CoA is preferentially used as a primer, in comparison to acetyl CoA, in fatty acid synthesis.

In spite of this evidence that C_2 units are combined to make C_4, presumably by both the malonyl CoA pathway and preferentially by the β-reduction mechanism of Lin and Kumar, and despite demonstration that C_4 units entering mammary tissue are in significant proportion degraded to C_2 units,[220] there must not be complete equilibration of all these metabolites. The data of Walker et al.[368] showed clearly that ^{14}C-acetate injected intravenously or infused into the mammary gland of the lactating goat does not proportionately label the C_4–C_8 milk fatty acids to the degree it does the C_{10}–C_{14} acids. This effect has been observed in previous studies of Popjak et al.[296] and of Lawrence and Hawke.[212] Thus there must be a blood source of carbon in addition to acetate for synthesis of the C_4–C_8 milk fatty acids. Ahrens and Luick[4] have shown that a C_4 unit can be used intact in the synthesis of the short-chain fatty acids of milk fat. These various findings suggest that β-hydroxybutyrate from the blood is an important source of carbon for the C_4–C_8 milk fatty acids and that it may be used intact to some extent for this purpose. This contention is confirmed by the experiments of McCarthy and Smith.[239] Their research clarifies the matter considerably by showing that the avidin-insensitive pathway of cow mammary tissue involves incorporation of acetate into C_4–C_8 fatty acids and of β-hydroxybutyrate into C_4 fatty acid. The acetate pathway in question was found to reside at least in part in the mitochondrion, while that for β-hydroxybutyrate to butyrate was found in the supernatant (cytoplasm) fraction. In parallel studies with rat mammary tissue, utilization of acetate and β-hydroxybutyrate was small and confined to the supernatant fraction. β-hydroxybutyrate was broken down to C_2 units before incorporation.

Another source of carbon for the synthesis of milk fatty acids and particularly for butyrate has been demonstrated by Dimick et al.[84] Infusion of 1-^{14}C laurate into the mammary gland of the lactating goat was seen to label the C_4 in particular and to a much lesser extent the other C_6–C_{16} fatty acids of the milk fat. The quantitative significance of this path is not known, but may be small since normally little oxidation of long-chain fatty acids appears to occur in ruminant mammary tissue.[8]

In summary, acetate and β-hydroxybutyrate supply carbon for synthesis of ruminant milk fatty acids (C_4–C_{16}) via the malonyl CoA pathway. This pathway accounts for only part of the C_{16} and little if any of the C_{18} fatty acids. Moreover, it appears to account for only a small portion of the C_4–C_8 fatty acids. These latter derive substantially from β-hydroxybutyrate and acetate by other pathways, one of which is associated with the mitochondrion. These pathways are so-called avidin-insensitive. Glucose, as opposed to acetate or β-hydroxybutyrate, is the prime substrate for milk fatty acid synthesis in the rat. This variation in substrate utilization appears to be an important reason for differences in milk fatty acid composition between ruminants and non-ruminants.

3. δ-hydroxy- and β-keto-fatty acids

There is an interesting series of δ-hydroxy- and β-keto-fatty acids in ruminant milk fats. The principal members of the series correspond to milk fatty acids with even numbers of carbons from C_6 through C_{16} (see composition of milk lipids). The metabolic significance of these acids is uncertain. At the moment they seem best viewed as side products of milk fatty acid synthesis. Dimick et al.[84] proposed δ-oxidation of fatty acids as a plausible mechanism to explain the origin of δ-hydroxy fatty acids. In ^{14}C-acetate labeling experiments[352,368] with the intact goat the δ-hydroxy acids exhibited specific activities slightly lower but closely correlated with the activity of their corresponding non-hydroxylated fatty acids. However, Swenson et al.[352] have since indicated that no δ-hydroxy acids could be demonstrated in milk fat following infusion of ^{14}C-labeled decanoic or dodecanoic acids into the mammary gland of the lactating goat.

In contrast to the δ-hydroxy acids, the β-keto acids exhibited in in vivo labeling experiments somewhat higher specific activities than their corresponding unsubstituted milk fatty acids of the same chain lengths.[212] This would indicate that the keto acids are intermediates in fatty acid synthesis rather than of fatty acid degradation.

It was shown some years ago at our laboratory and those of Unilever Ltd. that the δ-lactones and methyl ketones derived from the corresponding oxygenated fatty acids are of considerable importance in the flavor of milk and milk products (see reviews 85, 102, 193). Under processing and storage conditions the β-keto acids rearrange to methyl ketones and the δ-hydroxy acids to δ-lactones.

It is probable that the number of fatty acids present in milk fat is only limited by the sensitivity of current methods of detection and involves rather large statistical possibilities. We have discussed some of the better known and gross components in this section. Information on additional components is given in the following section on milk lipid composition (Section V).

4. Pattern of milk fatty acids

The distinguishing consideration concerning fatty acid synthesis in mammary tissue is not so much the functioning of classical pathways as it is the regulatory mechanisms that produce the unique patterns of fatty acid chain lengths in the milk triglycerides. It is adequately demonstrated that fatty acid synthetase accomplishes the condensation of C_2 units in mammary tissue as it does in other tissues and cells. The principal and virtually exclusive product under optimum in vitro reaction conditions is palmitate. Smith[339] has shown that fatty acid synthetase of liver and of mammary gland are very similar, if not identical and that they produce one and the same product, palmitate, under the same conditions. However, each mammalian species produces its own pattern of milk fatty acids, and ruminant milk fats are remarkable for containing substantial levels of C_4, C_6 and C_8 fatty acids (see preceding) Other species have their variations, C_8 and C_{10}, in the rabbit for example, and many have significant quantities of C_{10}, C_{12} and C_{14}. So these acids are produced by regulation of the malonyl CoA pathway and/or other pathways involved.

Prolactin action in mammary tissue apparently is essential in inducing the characteristic pattern of milk fatty acids.[351] In the bovine a comparison of mammary tissue 1–2 weeks prepartum with that 2 days prepartum demonstrated a dramatic development of capability for milk fatty acid and triglyceride synthesis just prior to parturition.[191]

The nature of milk fatty acids that are made is intimately related to triglyceride synthesis. More particularly the synthesis of fatty acids in the cytoplasm seems regulated in some manner by triglyceride synthesis on the endoplasmic reticulum. It is known that perfused udders, tissue slices[20] and even isolated mammary cells[184,186,192] will produce the appropriate pattern of milk fatty acids, but that cell-free homogenates will not. Thus the regulation must be in the intact cell. If the short-chain acids are being produced by mitochondria, juxtaposition of the latter to the site of triglyceride synthesis may be required. Perhaps it is more than coincidental that mitochondria are frequently seen abutting milk fat droplets in the cell. An ubiquitous protein which binds long-chain fatty acids in the cytosol has been reported,[260] and evidence that binding proteins for milk fatty acids might regulate their chain lengths has been communicated by S. Smith (unpublished). Undoubtedly a most important regulator of milk fatty acid chain lengths results from cellular requirements for milk fat droplet formation. The fatty acids which are used are those meeting these requirements, and synthesis of those which do not might be inhibited by feedback. This problem leads logically to a consideration of triglyceride synthesis which follows.

D. *Triglyceride synthesis*

In considering the mechanisms of milk triglyceride synthesis the cytological aspect is important (see Section III C, Fat). In essence this involves accumulation of triglycerides synthesized on the endoplasmic reticulum into droplets. For triglyceride accumulation to continue in an orderly fashion and for secretion to be facilitated a liquid condition in the fat droplet is required. The availability of butyric and oleic acids, and perhaps the C_6 and C_8 acids as well, would tend to determine liquidity and would be rate-limiting in triglyceride synthesis under conditions of ruminant mammary metabolism. In monogastrics where supply of unsaturated acids to the mammary gland is relatively abundant or in ruminants where polyunsaturates are protected from rumen hydrogenation, oleate and butyrate probably would not influence the rate of milk triglyceride synthesis. The high level, roughly 70 mole %, of C_8 and C_{10} fatty acids contained in rabbit milk fat indicates regulation of fatty acid synthetase by the requirement to produce liquid triglycerides. This is not in contradiction to the proposal by Carey and Dils[59,60] that malonyl CoA supply or acetyl CoA carboxylase activity may regulate chain length. In fact the many interrelated reactions in triglyceride synthesis starting with acetate, β-hydroxybutyrate and glucose and the many aspects of cellular machinery involved suggest that no single factor explains the pattern of fatty acids in the milk triglycerides of a particular species.

A class of enzymes that has received limited study and is indispensable in the synthesis of the milk triglycerides is the acyl transferases. The transferase which moves the palmitoyl group from its CoA ester to glycerolphosphate in guinea pig mammary tissue has been investigated by Kuhn.[200,201] He observed that this enzyme is bound to the endoplasmic reticulum and that it increases 37-fold in specific activity at parturition. Kuhn defends the possibility that this enzyme is rate-limiting in the synthesis of milk triglycerides, pointing out that crucial substrates such as glycerolphosphate and long-chain acyl CoA are not. Whether there are many transferase enzymes in mammary tissue with a high degree of specificity for chain length and/or unsaturation of acyl groups and for accepting substrate hydroxyls is not known. A further question is the relative ease with which these enzymes utilize CoA esters as compared with acyl carrier protein (of fatty acid synthetase) as substrate.

Another enzyme which increases many-fold at parturition and which must have gate-like qualities in milk triglyceride synthesis is lipoprotein lipase.[94,233,307] Mendelson and Scow[241] indicate that this enzyme may regulate uptake of serum triglycerides in mammary tissue and this would in turn determine the supply of long-chain acids, particularly C_{18} acids, for milk triglyceride synthesis.

1. Glycerol-3-phosphate pathway

The most ubiquitous known biochemical route in the synthesis of triglycerides is that involving glycerol-3-phosphate. According to the Kennedy scheme[180,371] this compound, generated either by glycolysis or the action of glycerol kinase, is acylated with 2 moles of fatty acid to yield the sn-1,2 diacyl phosphatidic acid, which in turn is converted by phosphatidic acid phosphohydrolase to a diglyceride. This latter compound then is acylated with a third mole of fatty acid to yield the triglyceride (Fig. 17). Since the experiments of Luick,[225] it has been known that glucose is converted to milk triglyceride glycerol in the bovine mammary gland. However, the demonstration of phosphatidic acid, a key intermediate in the Kennedy scheme, in either milk or mammary tissue has proven difficult. A number of complicating factors have contributed to this problem. Under normal conditions there appears to be essentially no mass

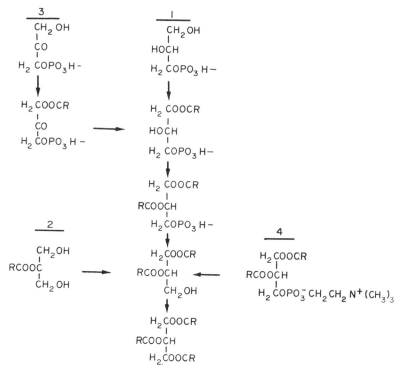

FIG. 17. Proposed routes in the biosynthesis of milk triglycerides. (1) glycerol-3-phosphate pathway, (2) 2-monoglyceride pathway, (3) 1-hydroxyacetetone-3-phosphate pathway, and (4) reversal of phosphatidylcholine synthesis.

of this compound in either milk or mammary tissue. Our observations in this connection are confirmed by Kuhn[201] who could not qualitatively detect phosphatidic acid in guinea pig mammary tissue. A number of phosphatidic acid preparations we have obtained from supply houses appeared to be methyl phosphatidates, as a result of extracting preparative reactions (phosphatidylcholine plus phospholipase D) with solvents containing methanol (see Yang et al.[385]) rather than authentic phosphatidic acid. This has created confusion regarding the behavior of the compound in thin-layer chromatographic systems. Few authors have given adequate details as to their methods of isolating phosphatidic acid. Under some circumstances phosphatidic acid is generated from diglyceride.[58] In addition, phosphatidic acid is always a potential artifact by decomposition of any of the other glycerolphospholipids.

The glycerol-3-phosphate pathway has been demonstrated in mammary tissue *in vitro*.[80,200,234,300] Supporting evidence has also been provided for its existence in mammary cell preparations[185] and in freshly secreted milk.[187] We have demonstrated phosphatidic acid, the key intermediate of this pathway, in the intact rat mammary gland; a representative experimental result is presented in Fig. 18. It shows that a very high specific activity component that coincides precisely in two-dimensional TLC systems with phosphatidic acid is detectable in mammary tissue within a few minutes following intravenous injection of $H_3{}^{32}PO_4$ into the rat.

2. Monoglyceride pathway

It has been shown that triglyceride synthesis in intestinal mucosa involves monoglyceride as substrate.[327] Monoglycerides and fatty acids released by lipase in the lumen of the intestine are transported into the mucosal cells and are there resynthesized into triglycerides. This synthesis requires prior activation of the fatty acids by adenosine triphosphate and coenzyme A. McBride and Korn[235] have provided evidence of such a monoglyceride pathway in guinea pig mammary tissue *in vitro*. On the basis of the positioning of palmitic acid in high and low molecular weight milk triglycerides, Dimick et al.[81] have noted that the 2-position of the high molecular weight fraction appears to be occupied by a palmitate precursor from the blood. Yet when ^{14}C-palmitic acid is given intravenously (goat) it preferentially labels the 1- or 3-positions. This suggests that something other than serum fatty acid in free form, such as would be produced by lipoprotein lipase activity in capillaries of mammary tissue, accounts for the observations of Dimick et al.[81] They proposed that a 2-monoglyceride is responsible for this positioning effect.

Recently Coccodrilli[68] has shown that milk triglyceride glycerol derived from glucose within the mammary gland (goat) is diluted in the high molecular weight fraction by glycerol from another source (Fig. 19). It appears beyond doubt that at least part of this other source is derived from blood triglycerides through action of lipoprotein lipase. It is known that lactating mammary tissue contains glycerol kinase,[234] and this enzyme has been demonstrated in freshly secreted bovine milk.[187] The question seems to be whether the serum triglycerides utilized in the synthesis of milk fat are only partially degraded to an extent that considerable monoglyceride remains or whether there is total breakdown to free fatty acids and glycerol. West et al.[373] prepared goat chylomicrons with double labeling of the triglycerides using duodenal infusion of ^{14}C-glycerol tripalmitate and 9,10-$^3H_2$ palmitic acid. The preparation was infused into

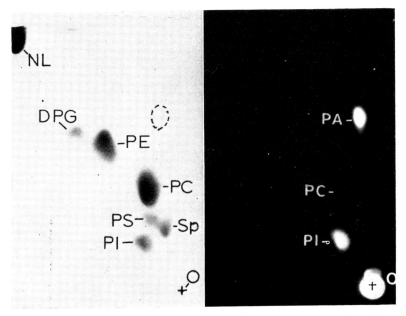

FIG. 18. Left: thin-layer chromatographic separation of polar lipids extracted from lactating rat mammary gland 10 min following i.v. injection of 0.2 mCi of $H_3{}^{32}PO_4$. Right: autoradiogram of the same thin-layer separation showing location of radioactivity (^{32}P) in various lipids. Abbreviations: NL, neutral lipids; DPG, diphosphatidylglycerol; PE, phosphatidylethanolamine; PA, phosphatidic acid (position of PA mass where indicated by broken line); PC, phosphatidylcholine; PS, phosphatidylserine; PI, phosphatidylinositol; Sp, sphingomyelin; O, origin. (Patton[269]).

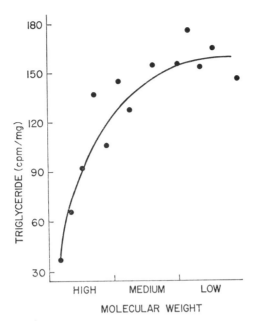

Fig. 19. Specific activity in glycerol of fractionated triglycerides of goat milk following intramammary infusion with U-^{14}C-glucose (Coccodrilli[68]).

the mammary artery of a second goat and the milk fat triglycerides were analyzed for ^{14}C/^{3}H ratio. It was found that the ratio dropped to 0.65 in the milk triglyceride as compared to the unity value in the infused chylomicrons. This certainly implies some degree of hydrolysis of plasma triglycerides taken up by mammary tissue in synthesis of milk triglycerides. West et al. concluded that the hydrolysis was extensive or complete. On the other hand, since released glycerol is water-soluble and would be expected to move and be metabolized in quite different ways than released fatty acid, one might conclude that the ratio of 0.65 indicates considerable structural integrity of the plasma glycerides was maintained in transfer to milk triglycerides. Bickerstaffe et al.[27] using intravenous glycerol monoether infusions have shown that a 2-monoether is incorporated into milk triglycerides. This implies that a 2-monoglyceride would be metabolized similarly provided that it was not hydrolyzed first. Perfusion experiments with rat mammary gland have established that lipolysis of serum triglycerides occurs outside the blood stream and confirm that products of the lipolysis (glycerol and free fatty acid) are returned in substantial proportion to the blood as well as retained by the tissue.[241] Using a similar double labeling approach in these experiments to the one employed by West et al., Mendelson and Scow[241] found that tissue triglycerides exhibited essentially the same fatty acid to glycerol labeling ratio as that of the chylomicrons. Recent research by Polheim et al.[294] suggests that 2-monoglycerides have an inhibiting effect on the glycerol-3-phosphate pathway of triglyceride synthesis in adipose and intestinal tissues, In addition, monoglycerides have been reported unable to serve as acyl acceptors in the presence of mammary gland preparations from the rat[80] and goat.[300] This is in contrast to the findings of McBride and Korn[235] with the guinea pig and somewhat surprising since ethanol is a ready acyl (palmitoyl) acceptor even in fresh milk.[280]

In any event, unequivocal evidence that a 2-monoglyceride pathway either does or does not exist *in vivo* for the synthesis of milk fat triglycerides is yet forthcoming. It does appear, however, that by some selective mechanism palmitate in the 2-position of serum triglycerides is directed to the 2-position in milk triglycerides.

3. *Other pathways*

We have postulated a pathway of milk triglyceride synthesis involving phosphatidylcholine as an intermediate.[284] It is known that the preponderant phospholipid in the forming milk fat droplet is phosphatidylcholine, which is presumed to occur at the droplet periphery.[140,272,273] We have suggested that a diglyceride moiety derived from this phospholipid may serve as an acceptor of short-chain acyl groups, particularly butyrate, in the synthesis of milk fat triglycerides. The limited evidence for such a pathway stems from a variety of lipid-labeling experiments[190,275,281,283] in which it has been observed that phosphatidylcholine of mammary tissue and milk is promptly and intensely labeled. Since phosphatidylcholine enters milk at the same rate and in roughly the same amount as phosphatidylethyanolamine, one is challenged to account for the metabolic activity of the former. The existence of the pathway in question (i.e., phosphatidylcholine $\longrightarrow$ diglyceride $\longrightarrow$ triglyceride) has been demonstrated in rat liver[162] and is in essence a back reaction of the enzyme systems which synthesizes phosphatidylcholine.

Another explanation of turnover in labeling of phosphatidylcholine with ^{14}C-fatty acid, but not with $H_3{}^{32}PO_4$, is that the phospholipid is an intermediate in fatty acid transport. Wright and Green[382] have shown that incubation of rat liver cells with ^{14}C-fatty acid witnesses incorporation of the tracer into phosphatidylcholine of the plasma membrane even before its incorporation into phosphatidic acid. They propose that this reflects a mechanism whereby fatty acid is transported into the cell.

Hajra and Agranoff[124] propose that 1-hydroxyacetone-3-phosphates may provide a unique pathway in the synthesis of glycerides and phosphoglycerides in which the one and two positions would be differentially specified. There has been no investigation of the possible existence of this pathway in lactating mammary tissue. The four pathways to triglycerides discussed here are summarized schematically in Fig. 17.

4. *Properties of the triglycerides*

The composition of milk triglycerides is dealt with in Section V. We would like to mention here a few interesting characteristics about composition in relation to synthesis and degradation of the triglycerides. Since butyrate occurs at a level of about 10 mole % in ruminant milk fats and only one mole per mole of triglyceride, a substantial fraction of the total triglycerides are monobutyryl.[83,228,290] The C_6 and C_8 acids also tend to occur one mole per mole of triglyceride[228] so, in all, roughly half of the triglyceride molecules contain two long-chain acyl groups (C_{16} and C_{18}) and one short-chain (C_4–C_8). The remainder is composed of all long-chain acyl groups. On thin-layer chromatography the milk fat triglycerides show a distinct tendency to separate into two spots, the leading one of which is composed of only long-chain acyl derivatives and the trailing one which contains the long- and short-chain acids.[258] Kuksis and his associates,[202–204] in developing gas chromatography technique for the direct separation of glycolipids, have produced elegant separations of triglycerides by aggregate numbers of acyl carbons. Ruminant milk fat by this method of analysis

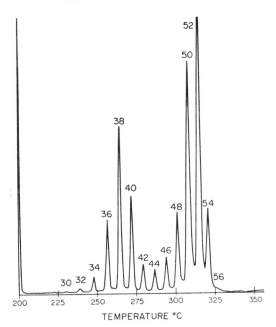

FIG. 20. Temperature programmed gas–liquid chromatogram of bovine milk triglycerides. Numbering corresponds to total number of acyl carbons in triglyceride molecules of that peak (Kuksis and Breckenridge[203]).

shows two families of peaks based on total acyl carbons per triglyceride: one centered in the 36, 38 and 40 region containing one short-chain acid with two long chains and the other from 48 through 54 involving only long chains (Fig. 20). Because of a lack of short-chain acids, triglycerides from human and most other milks do not show this pattern (see ref. 203).

Considering the chain length and unsaturation of fatty acids plus their positioning on the glycerol, it is possible to make an analytical approach to the highly complex problem of milk glycerolipid composition. For discussion of methods and results in this area see Section V.

Because of the short-chain acids in ruminant milk fats (i.e., butyric, caproic, caprylic, etc.) enzymatic hydrolysis produces a powerful aroma which may be desirable or unpleasant depending upon circumstances. With respect to the aroma of certain cheeses the release of these acids is indispensable. On the other hand stools and stomach rejecta of babies fed cow's milk ordinarily have this aroma in an unpleasant degree and context. Breast fed babies are not subject to the odor because these acids are essentially absent from human milk fat.

E. *Synthesis of phospholipids and glycolipids*

The phospholipids and glycolipids of milk are associated largely or exclusively with membrane vesicles in the skim milk phase or membrane surrounding milk fat globules. These membranes were structural elements of the cell and there is no reason to believe that the phospholipids of the lactating cell are synthesized by different pathways or mechanisms than those for milk. In essence, some of the machinery of the cell (membranes, enzymes, etc.) continuously passes into the milk. As shown by Parsons and Patton,[265] there are essentially identical polar lipids in cow's milk and mammary tissue, the main difference being in their proportions (Fig. 21). The principal polar lipid-bearing material in the tissue is endoplasmic reticulum which is mainly rich in phosphatidylcholine and phosphatidylethanolamine; whereas the source of polar lipid in milk is primarily plasma membrane which contains substantial sphingomyelin and cerebrosides compared to the tissue polar lipids. A further difference is that the latter contain about 3% cardiolipin of mitochondrial origin. Since mitochondria are effectively retained in the cell,[274] there is virtually no cardiolipin in milk. Beside the membrane material in milk, one other likely source of polar lipids exists and that is the surface layer which the milk fat globule had within the cell just prior to secretion. At secretion this surface is overlaid with plasma membrane.

1. *Phospholipids*

The studies of Easter *et al.*[88] indicate that most, if not all, the phospholipids of milk are synthesized *de novo* in mammary tissue. This results from evidence that intravenously administered $^{32}P_i$ labels (goat) milk phospholipids more promptly and intensely than it labels blood serum phospholipids and that autoradiograms from such experiments reveal all the milk phospholipids to be labeled approximately in proportion to their masses. Further, in $^{32}P_i$ experiments with both the rat and the goat, the ratios between masses for total milk phosphorus and milk lipid phosphorus and ratios of their total radioactivities were essentially identical, which suggests that inorganic phosphorus and lipid phosphorus of milk were being derived from a single pool of phosphate within the gland. An additional observation from the study was that no dietary phospholipid (U-^{14}C-phosphatidylcholine) was transferred intact into rat milk. The capacity of isolated mammary cells to synthesize the glycerophospholipids of milk has been demonstrated using radioactive glycerol.[185] Annison *et al.*[8] found no arteriovenous difference in serum phospholipids across the lactating mammary gland of the goat. This supports the contention that these lipids are not taken up from the blood and that milk phospholipids are synthesized *de novo* in the mammary tissue.

While it seems safe to conclude that the milk phospholipids are substantially if not completely synthesized in the mammary gland, there has not yet been sufficiently rigorous research to preclude the possibility that some species of milk phospholipid in some degree originates from the circulation. A scheme outlining biosynthetic pathways for the major glycerophospholipids of bovine milk is shown in Fig. 22. The other principal phospholipid of milk and mammary tissue is sphingomyelin. Its synthesis involves the formation of ceramide (N-acyl sphingosine) from sphingosine and acyl CoA and presumably the reaction of the ceramide with CDP-choline. However, recent reports (see Addendum) that the phosphoryl choline group of sphingomyelin can be derived from phosphatidylcholine are pertinent.

From experience with thin-layer chromatographic separations of phospholipids from milk and mammary tissue of various species, we suspect that phosphatidylglycerol is present in tissue at levels of a percent or so of total lipid phosphorus. No doubt traces of other phospholipids are regularly or transiently present also, but

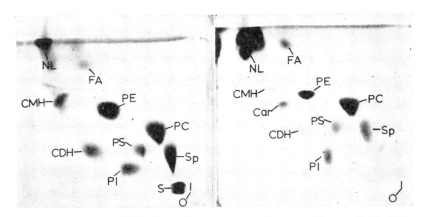

FIG. 21. Two-dimensional thin-layer chromatograms of bovine milk polar lipids (left) and mammary tissue total lipids (right). The chromatograms were developed from right to left with chloroform–methanol–water–28% aqueous ammonia 130:70:8:0.5 and then upwards with chloroform–acetone–methanol–acetic acid–water 100:40:20:20:10. Spots were detected by chromic acid spray and charring. O, origin; S, carbohydrate (lactose) and protein; Sp, sphingomyelin; PC, phosphatidyl choline; PS, phosphatidylserine; PI, phosphatidyl inositol; PE, phosphatidyl ethanolamine; Car, cardiolipin; CDH, ceramide dihexoside; CMH, ceramide monohexoside; FA, free fatty acid; NL, neutral lipid. (Adapted from Patton et al.[274])

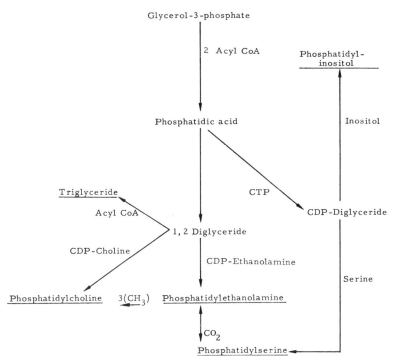

FIG. 22. Pathways in the biosynthesis of major glycerolipids occurring in milk and mammary tissue. CDP, cytodine diphosphate; CTP, cytodine triphosphate. (Adapted from schemes of Kennedy.[180])

characterization of these remains a challenge. The evidence regarding synthesis of phospholipids in various cell and tissue types points rather consistently to the endoplasmic reticulum as the site. Cardiolipin is a special consideration in that it is made by the mitochondrion,[78,141] and mitochondria of mammary tissue are rich in cardiolipin.[142,274] According to Hostetler et al.,[141] cardiolipin (diphosphatydylglycerol) is synthesized by the inner membrane of the mitochondrion from rat liver. The reaction is:

Phosphatidylglycerol + CDP diglyceride → diphosphatidylglycerol + CMP

It is highly probable that this is the pathway for synthesis of cardiolipin in mammary tissue. Since phosphatidylglycerol is a reactant, its presence in the tissue is predicted. The Golgi apparatus apparently does not synthesize glycerolipids according to studies with subcellular fractions of livers.[363] The plasma membrane of course is an unlikely site for synthesis of most cell phospholipid because it has at best only 1 or 2% of the total phospholipid in a cell such as the hepatocyte or mammary cell. There is no reason to believe that the phospholipids of milk and mammary tissue involve biosynthetic pathways that are different from those generally established for mammalian tissues. The reader is referred to the treatise edited by Ansell et al.[9] for a current and extensive review of the phospholipids.

In addition to the classic glycerophospholipids, small amounts of their plasmalogen analogues also occur in milk. Further information on proportions and fatty acid composition of phospholipids in milk are given in Section V.

2. Glycolipids

The two classes of glycolipids known to occur in milk and mammary tissue are the cerebrosides and gangliosides. A number of investigations have confirmed that cow's and goat's milks contain two principal cerebrosides (see review in ref. 166). These are glucosyl- and lactosyl-N-acyl sphingosines. At times a third component, apparently a trihexoside ceramide, is faintly evident on thin-layer chromatograms of milk polar lipids. The cerebrosides are associated with the membrane material in milk and are partitioned about 2:1 or 1:1 in association with fat globules and skim milk respectively. The distribution is similar to that of the phospholipids. The concentration of total cerebrosides in cows and goats milk is of the order of 20 to 50 mg/l.[166] Recently ceramide (N-acyl sphingosine) was isolated from bovine milk at a level of 2.2 mg/l by Fujino and Fujishima.[110] They found that sphingomyelin, cerebroside and ceramide from milk have very similar fatty acid compositions. Morrison and Hay[248] have observed very similar long-chain base composition in sphingomyelin and cerebrosides of milk. This supports the concept of a common precursor of these lipids; presumably the same ceramide molecules (on the same side of the membrane) are substrate for both cerebrosides and sphingomyelin synthesis. Kayser and Patton[166] noted reduced levels of the C_{22}–C_{24} fatty acids characteristic of the milk cerebrosides in the cerebrosides of the skim milk phase. The bovine serum cerebrosides are relatively devoid of these long-chain acids,[336] which raises the possibility that serum cerebrosides may gain entry to skim milk. Retention of sphingolipids in membranes may depend on their containing long-chain fatty acids (C_{20}–C_{25}). We have postulated that formation of plasma membrane involves preferential retention of sphingolipids.[283]

Gangliosides, glycosphingolipids containing sialic acid, have been detected in bovine mammary tissue and milk[145,167,171] (see also ref 48, p. 108). In the latter medium they appear to be concentrated in the milk fat globule membrane. The cerebrosides are substrates in sequential enzymatic steps whereby the gangliosides are synthesized.[309] Glycosyltransferase enzymes which accomplish the glycosylation of lipids and proteins appear to be concentrated in the Golgi membranes.[167,173,174,243] This is consistent with the antigenic properties of the glycoproteins and glycolipids and with their occurrence on the outer surface of the plasma membrane. The inner surface of Golgi membranes becomes the outer surface of the cell by virtue of secretory vesicle emptying. However, Keenan et al. provide evidence that a substantial fraction of total ganglioside occurs in the endomembranes of rat liver and bovine mammary gland[171] and that gangliosides of mammary tissue are synthesized in the Golgi apparatus.[167] Information on the nature, amounts and distribution of gangliosides in milk and mammary tissue is limited. This may change in light of recent interest in the possible function of gangliosides in contact inhibition of mammary cell replication.[171,173] Breast cancer involves unbridled multiplication of transformed mammary epithelial cells.

F. Cholesterol

Despite the strong public interest in cholesterol because of the diet–heart issue, the information available on cholesterol in milk is somewhat limited. We will review and discuss basic functions and metabolism of cholesterol, the amounts and forms of cholesterol in milk and the origins of milk cholesterol. Some practical considerations regarding cholesterol in milk are presented subsequently in this section.

1. *Functions and metabolism of cholesterol*

Membrane structure and function, serum lipoprotein metabolism, and aging of arteries (atherosclerosis) overlap in the central consideration of cholesterol metabolism. The principles that govern cholesterol metabolism by mammary tissue are not fundamentally different from those involved in other structures of the body and there may be a unique advantage in studying the mammary system as a model of cholesterol metabolism. Milk provides a physiological and ultrastructural record as how cholesterol entering or synthesized within the body is transported. As discussed subsequently, cholesterol fed to an animal finds its way to membranes of the lactating cell and into milk.

While cholesterol function at the molecular level is the subject currently of intensive research, several properties of the molecule are notable: (1) In monolayers films of phospholipids the addition of cholesterol tends to contract the surface area of the monolayer (see review by van Deenan[361] on phospholipids and membranes). This might be stated more generally that cholesterol tends to facilitate packing of lipid molecules in a membrane. (2) In a bilayer membrane, cholesterol tends to render the interior (non-polar area) of the bilayer more uniformly liquid by binding most strongly to the region in lipid molecules close to polar head groups, roughly carbons 1–7 in the fatty acid chains.[311] (3) In comparison to cholesterol esters, free cholesterol promotes formation of lipid bilayers while cholesterol esters promote lipid droplets. (4) Cholesterol appears to accumulate in cell membrane as an aging phenomenon. Evidence for the latter two propositions is presented subsequently.

These principles regarding behavior and properties of the cholesterol molecule may provide insight to its transport. For example, if cholesterol tends to accumulate on one side of a bilayer, thus producing closer packing of the lipids on that side, the circumstances for vesiculation of the membrane may thereby be facilitated; i.e., one side of the membrane would shrink in comparison to the other side thus producing an invagination. If the outer cholesterol-rich surface of the membrane contained factors promotive of fusion, such as a catalytic protein, relatively weak surface charge, etc., the vesiculation (endocytosis) might be completed placing the vesicle of surface membrane and its extracellular contents inside the cell. The fate of such a vesicle might involve lysis within the cell, fusion with the internal membranes of the cell or passage through the cell. Portman and Alexander[298] report a prominent change with age and early atherogenesis in the arterial intima of the primate (squirrel monkey) is a proliferation of plasma membrane in the form of many vesicles. Portman[297] suggests that a mechanism of the type described may account for this phenomenon. In this instance a serum lipoprotein may be conceived as transferring cholesterol to the membrane lining the blood vessel and this enrichment may trigger the pinocytotic process. While such a mechanism is only hypothetically established, we view it as being potentially of very broad significance not only in atherogenesis or cholesterol transport but in pinocytotic phenomena in general.

The postulated mechanism whereby cholesterol maintains fluidity in the non-polar region of a membrane may be of particular importance in establishing membrane lipid transition temperature from liquid to solid below normal body temperature, even though the membrane were composed of saturated lipids. This might be particularly important in ruminants whose lipids are relatively saturated, and it may be quite relevant in membranes of mammals in which conditions might lead to oxidative deterioration of polyunsaturated lipids (lungs, blood vessels, etc.)

Concerning the comparative effects of free and esterified cholesterol on structure, investigations of the ultrastructure of serum lipoproteins in sickness and health have produced interesting evidence. It has been observed that a deficiency of the enzyme lecithin-cholesterol acyl-transferase (LCAT) in human serum is associated with an abnormal (non-globular) structure of the serum high density lipoprotein (HDL) in which the lipids are disposed in multilayers.[105,126] The appearance under the electron microscope of this HDL is aptly described as resembling stacks of poker chips. This observation is intriguing because the essential difference in composition which appears to induce the change in structure involves whether the cholesterol is esterified.

The LCAT enzyme transfers the fatty acid in the 2-position of phosphatidylcholine to cholesterol. This esterification of cholesterol promotes a globular structure of the HDL while the absence of esterified cholesterol, LCAT deficiency, induces the multilayered configuration. Measurements of these layers by Forte et al.[105] indicated the thickness of the repeating unit to be 50–55 Å, which agrees with the thickness observed for bimolecular layers of lipids in membranes.[14] A fact of further interest is that lipid droplets in atheromatous plaques appear to be virtually pure cholesterol ester deposits.[207]

It is worth considering the relative metabolic significance of lipids deposited in a membrane and those in a droplet. The arrangement of lipid molecules in a bilayer assures their accessibility to the cytoplasm so that enzymatic transformation in the membrane or transport from the membrane is theoretically possible for all molecules. On the other hand, the formation of a globular structure facilitates the submergence of highly non-polar molecules such as cholesterol esters into the interior of the lipid phase, thus rendering them more inaccessible to degradation or removal. As a consequence, droplets are logical storage forms and considerations of liquidity and molecular accessibility are pertinent to the formation and degration of milk fat droplets.

It seems to be intuitive in the thinking of many lipid biochemists that cholesterol can be something of a metabolic clinker; i.e., because of its structural stability and relative unreactivity that it may tend to remain or accumulate when other types of molecules have long since turned over. Some evidence[267] supporting this notion has been gathered at our laboratory. If from the information in the literature one plots the concentration of cholesterol and sphingomyelin as a function of total lipids in membranes of the rat hepatocyte, one finds that their concentrations are positively correlated and tend to be highest in the plasma membrane (Fig. 23). In the membrane systems of the hepatocyte the plasma membrane contains the highest concentration of lipid (40–50%) so that the actual amounts of both cholestrol and sphingomyelin are 4 to 6 times as high in the plasma membrane in comparison to the endoplasmic reticulum. In the case of sphingomyelin we have presented evidence to show that once it is incorporated in the membrane it tends to remain there as compared to the other phospholipids (see Figs. 10, 11 and 12). The same appears true for cholesterol although direct evidence of this is yet forthcoming. As discussed elsewhere (Section III), a variety of findings supports the theory of membrane transformation and flow in secretory cells such as the hepatocyte and mammary cell. This theory postulates that

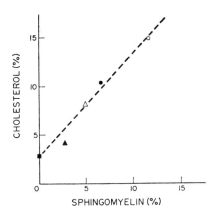

FIG. 23. The relationship (wt. %) between cholesterol and sphingomyelin in membranes of the rat hepatocyte. ■ mitochondrion, ▲ nucleus, △ endoplasmic reticulum, ● Golgi apparatus, ○ plasma membrane (Patton[267]).

the plasma membrane is an older phase of the cytoplasmic membranes and is derived from the endoplasmic reticulum via the Golgi apparatus. Endoplasmic reticulum is the site of cholesterol synthesis in the (liver) cell.[63]

The cholesterol in the blood serum is of particular interest because this is being conveyed all over the body and it is taken up by mammary tissue among others. One source of serum cholesterol is the diet. This has been demonstrated in various species of both lactating[67,69,87] and non-lactating animals.[73,152,353,376] A further point of interest is that the level of cholesterol in the human diet is positively correlated with the level in the serum.[232] Additional major sources are the intestinal mucosa and the liver. Both of these sites secrete cholesterol into the intestinal lumen and into the serum. The liver contributes cholesterol to the digesta in the form of bile and cholesterol in VLDLs to the blood. The intestinal mucosa secretes cholesterol into the lumen as well as taking it up from there, so that an equilibrium exists at that site. The intestinal mucosa deposits chylomicrons and VLDLs into lymph and these ultimately enter the circulation. It has been claimed that the intestine is the major site of cholesterol synthesis in the rat.[64] In the ruminant the diet being mainly if not exclusively plant material provides little or no cholesterol. However, rumen organisms, particularly protozoa, synthesize cholesterol which is metabolized when these organisms are digested. There may be some secretion of cholesterol into the rumen by the rumen epithelium and certainly sloughed tissue of the upper alimentary tract contributes some "dietary" cholesterol in the ruminant. The literature conveys the impression that cholesterol not only leaves the serum and penetrates tissues but that it leaves tissues and reenters blood.[297]

In addition to assimilation of dietary cholesterol, *de novo* synthesis of cholesterol in the various tissues of the body and its transport via the circulation, mammalian metabolism includes a number of routes for degradation and elimination of the compound These include oxidation to bile acids in the liver and elimination by the intestinal tract. Similarly, some cholesterol is secreted or sloughed with tissue into the intestinal tract and eliminated. Cholesterol is also converted to steroid hormones and waste products which are excreted in urine, sebum and perspiration. In order to contend with the complexities of cholesterol metabolism in man, some highly sophisticated models[117,317] have been devised toward the end of measuring the phenomena more precisely.

2. *Occurrence of cholesterol in milk*

While there seems to be little question that cholesterol occurs in milks of all mammalian species, as yet there have been no comparative studies. In fact the number of studies on ruminant milks, which are by far the ones most extensively consumed by humans, is small.

Cholesterol and cholesterol esters have been demonstrated in the milk lipids of the cow and goat.[278] The lipids were separated by column chromatography on silicic acid and the purified fractions of cholesterol esters identified by infrared spectrophotometry. This study indicated that cholesterol esters account for 10–15% of the cholesterol in milks of these species. De Man[76] observed this proportion to be 5–10% for bovine milk and a variety of products made from milk including cheddar cheese and butter. Cholesterol has also been analyzed in the milk of the rat,[67,87] rabbit[69] and guinea pig,[69] although these studies have been primarily concerned with origin of milk cholesterol.

The cholesterol and cholesterol esters of cow's and goat's milks occur both in association with milk fat globules and in the skim milk phase. In addition, fat globules may contain the two forms in the surface (membrane) layer as well as under this layer and in the case of the ester form in the globule core. The two fairly comprehensive analyses of cholesterol and cholesterol ester distribution in milk[146,250] have yielded conflicting results. From literature values and our own unpublished findings we conclude that *ca.* 20% of total cholesterol occurs in the skim milk phase, and the remainder is associated with the cream (milk fat globules) phase. Data regarding the amount and form of cholesterol associated with the core of fat globules pose difficulties because methods for partitioning the surface and cores of globules may easily lead to artifactual cholesterol distributions.

Cholesterol is known to exist in milk as a component of membranes. Plantz *et al.*[285,291,292] have shown that cholesterol is distributed in centrifuged skim milk in accord with phospholipid distribution and that both are concentrated in the membrane-rich fraction. The close correlation between the concentration of cholesterol and phospholipid in a series of hourly milkings from a goat is shown in Fig. 24. Similarly, the membrane of the milk fat globule, which represents plasma membrane from the lactating cell, is composed substantially of cholesterol and phospholipid. However, as discussed previously, cholesterol may occur in any or all of the compartments (core and several surfaces layers) of milk fat globule. If one considers that the cholesterol in milk tends to distribute itself approximately 80:20 between milk fat globules and skim milk phase while the phospholipids partitioning is about 60:40 it is obvious that the cholesterol/phospholipid ratio is considerably higher for milk fat globules than for membranes in the skim milk phase. Plantz *et al.* generally observed that cow's and goat's skim milk membrane fractions exhibited cholesterol/phospholipid molar ratios of 0.25–0.45. The ratio for fat globules was of the order of 1.0.

We reiterate that the number of comprehensive studies of cholesterol distribution, including forms of cholesterol and fatty acid composition of the esters, is quite small. Additional data seem needed on both ruminant and non-ruminant milks. Cholesterol

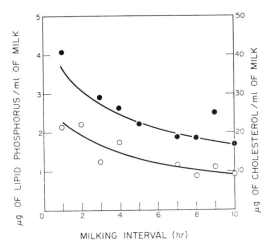

FIG. 24. Levels of lipid phosphorus (●) and total cholesterol (○) obtained in the skim milks from a series of hourly milkings of a goat initiated after normal twice daily milkings (Patton et al.[285]).

distribution data for milk from a single goat over a 13-day period are presented in Table 9. These data appear somewhat unique in that the esterified proportion is very low (2.6%) and the fraction of the total in the skim milk phase relatively high (34.3%), possibly because of inefficiency in removing cream (fat globules). We suspect that the trend shown in the table for ester cholesterol to account for a greater relative proportion of the total in the skim milk than in the fat globules is correct. Cholesterol is elevated in bovine colostrum.[139,354] The level falls from about 1.2% of total lipid in the first milk to a level of about 0.3–0.4% in several days[354] after which it slowly rises to the end of lactation.[139]

TABLE 9. *Cholesterol Distribution in Milk (Goat)*[a]

	Free		Esterified	
	Mean	Range	Mean	Range
Fat globules				
mg /100ml	8.49	4.76 – 12.37	0.15	0.09 – 0.30
%	65.7	48.5 – 81.0	42.2	19.9 – 58.7
Skim milk				
mg/100 ml	4.44	1.95 – 6.39	0.21	0.10 – 0.48
%	34.3	19.0 – 51.5	57.8	41.3 – 80.1
Whole milk				
mg/100 ml	12.93	8.80 – 17.79	0.36	0.20 – 0.59
%	97.4	94.8 – 98.4	2.6	1.6 – 5.2

[a] Data of Raphael et al. (see Addendum). Analysis of daily milkings for 13 days by the method of Searcy et al.[326]

3. *Origins of milk cholesterol*

Broadly there are three sources of the cholesterol in milk: the diet, the circulation and the mammary tissue. Cholesterol is synthesized from acetate by most if not all mammalian tissues. This was demonstrated for the mammary gland by Popjak and coworkers and has been confirmed for a number of species. The chemistry of the biosynthesis has been worked out largely by K. Bloch in the United States, Lynen in Germany and Popjak and Cornforth in England. The pathway (see the text by Lehninger[214]) involves condensations as follows: (C_2) $\longrightarrow$ mevalonate (C_5) $\longrightarrow$ geranyl pyrophosphate (C_{10}) $\longrightarrow$ farnesyl pyrophosphate (C_{15}) $\longrightarrow$ squalene (C_{30}). The latter aliphatic hydrocarbon undergoes cyclization, rearrangement and a number of additional reactions including decarboxylations to ultimately yield cholesterol ($C_{27}H_{46}O$). Chesterton[63] has shown that it is the endoplasmic reticulum which synthesizes cholesterol and cholesterol esters in the (rat) liver cell and it seems quite likely that this is the case for the lactating mammary cell. This implies that other cell membranes, which all contain cholesterol, derive from the endoplasmic reticulum.

In confirmation of earlier results[67,69,87] for the lactating rat, rabbit and guinea pig, data from our laboratory (manuscript in preparation) show clearly that ^{14}C-cholesterol placed in the abomasum (true stomach) of a goat is transported to her milk (Fig. 25). These data resemble closely those of Connor and Lin[69] for the guinea pig. We find in a second experiment, supporting data of Fig. 25, that several days after administering the tracer, free cholesterol in the milk fat globule and in the skim milk is of about the same order of specific activity. This is what would be expected if the dietary cholesterol equilibrated rather completely with membranes of the lactating cell.

Clarenburg and Chaikoff[67] interpret their data to mean that 11 % of milk cholesterol arises from the diet, and that about 80 % is synthesized *de novo* in mammary tissue. While contending that control or measurement of additional variables would be needed to assess the role of the liver and other serum lipoproteins, for purposes of

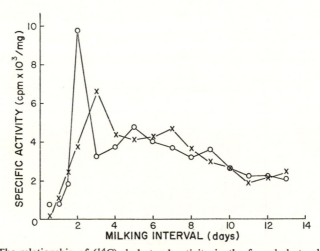

FIG. 25. The relationship of (^{14}C)-cholesterol activity in the free cholesterol of milk fat globules (○) and membrane material of skim milk (×) to milking times following the placing of 200 μCi of (^{14}C)-cholesterol in the abomasum of a lactating goat. Data by Raphael *et al.* (see Addendum).

calculation they assumed that liver contributes in a minor way to serum cholesterol and that chylomicrons are the principal donors of cholesterol from plasma to milk. The results of the study by Connor and Lin[69] do not easily lend themselves to a quantitative interpretation either. Their findings do confirm that the three sources (diet, serum and mammary tissue) contribute to milk cholesterol and that there is relatively greater transfer of serum cholesterol and less synthesis in the mammary tissue for the rabbit as compared to the guinea pig.

One of the major difficulties in these studies is the uncertainty as to which vehicle(s) in the blood are donating cholesterol to milk. If it were assumed in the Clarenburg and Chaikoff study that the vehicle in blood is representative of the entire serum cholesterol pool, then the dilution in activity from blood to milk is small (about 20%) and one can conclude that milk cholesterol is mainly (80%) derived from serum cholesterol. The serum vehicle(s) contributing cholesterol to milk may have cholesterol specific activities higher than that of the total serum and this would infer greater dilution by cholesterol arising in milk from synthesis in mammary tissue.

Recent studies at our laboratory have indicated that in the fasted rat all three serum lipoproteins (VLDL, LDL and HDL) can contribute cholesterol to milk and this tends to emphasize in our opinion the probable importance of HDLs in this regard. Earlier experiments by Evans and Patton[95] showed that the lower density (<1.063) bovine serum lipoproteins tended to transfer both cholesterol and cholesterol esters to HDLs during *in vitro* incubation. This makes it seem unlikely that transport of cholesterol from labeled HDLs to milk is by way of VLDLs or chylomicrons. However, that is not to say that the latter two serum components may not also donate cholesterol to milk. In essence then the first acceptor of dietary cholesterol is VLDLs in the intestinal mucosa. On entering the circulation these may transfer cholesterol to mammary tissue and to milk. They may also transfer cholesterol to LDLs and HDLs in the circulation and these may also transfer cholesterol to mammary tissue and to milk. Recent evidence by Eisenberg *et al.*[90,91] indicates that VLDLs are converted to LDLs and HDLs.

The data in Fig. 26 for labeling of esterified cholesterol in goat milk by dietary cholesterol is derived from the same samples as those for free cholesterol (Fig. 25). It will be evident that in comparison to the latter a completely different metabolism is being displayed for the cholesterol esters. They are an order of magnitude higher in specific activity, and in the case of the milk fat globule cholesterol esters a 2–4 day cyclic phenomenon is evident. These striking attributes were confirmed in a second experiment. It seems to be an unavoidable implication of these data that a major fraction of functional mammary cells were relatively unlabeled by serum ^{14}C cholesterol at the time another population of mammary cells were. A second deduction is that cholesterol esters of milk fat globules are being derived from a different pool of cholesterol than that supplying the free cholesterol. It is tempting to speculate that cholesterol esters are entering milk fat globules intact from the blood. According to Kinsella,[183] mammary cells in culture take up cholesterol esters intact. Since many other blood constituents gain entry to milk in one form or another, the possibility that cholesterol esters might do so is not unreasonable. A search in milk for HDLs which are rich in cholesterol esters might be rewarding. Since these particles might lodge in or transfer some of their constituents to membranes, perhaps a search for HDL

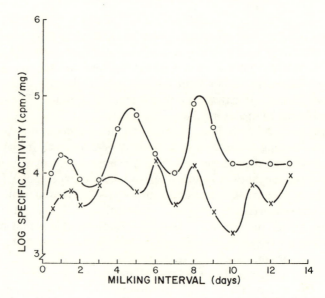

Fig. 26. Data, as in Fig. 25, for esterified cholesterol of milk fat globules (○) and skim milk membrane material (×).

protein components in milk membrane material with the aid of gel electrophoresis would be a useful approach.

In earlier studies at our laboratory[178,237,278] we noted that labeled fatty acids infused into the mammary gland of the lactating goat produced prompt and intense labeling of cholesterol esters of the milk. A recent investigation (T. W. Keenan and S. Patton, unpublished) has shown that this high intensity labeling which falls rapidly in successive milkings several hours after tracer injection is associated with cholesterol esters of the globule core. This was ascertained by analyzing activity of these esters in skim milk membrane, fat globules, fat globule membrane and fat globules less membrane. The labeling was found primarily in cholesterol esters of fat globule with or without membrane. The significance of this labeling is not known. It cannot be satisfactorily compared with labeling derived from dietary ^{14}C-cholesterol (Fig. 26) because the latter involved, among other differences, a much longer (13 days versus 1 day) observation period. As mentioned, the amount of cholesterol ester in milk is small, on the order of a few mg/l, and the possibility that traces of these esters are swept along with triglycerides into the gathering fat globule makes plausible the trapping of molecules with high radioactivity. On the other hand, this does not necessarily explain why the activity falls rapidly. The possibility exists that fatty acid is rapidly transferred through a cholesterol ester pool associated with synthesis of the milk fat droplet. The cholesterol esters of milk appear to exhibit an unusual metabolism and are worthy of further study.

G. Vitamin A

We have previously discussed the dietary component carotene (provitamin A) as an interesting marker of lipid metabolism which reaches milk in the cow but not the goat (p. 21). Vitamin A also may have unique characteristics in relation to the synthesis and secretion of milk. The occurrence and various factors influencing levels of vitamin A in milk have been reviewed by Hartman and Dryden.[130] Most milks are a fair to good source of vitamin A. The amount in milk of a given species varies with diet and fat content of the milk. The range is from 500 to 10,000 IU/l. The human and the cow average about 1500 to 2000 IU/l. Nearly all (94–98%) of the vitamin A in bovine milk occurs in the ester form. About 85% of the vitamin is associated with fat globules; the remainder is dispersed probably in association with membranes, in the skim milk. White et al.[374] have shown that vitamin A is distributed in fat globules in proportion to their surface area, as is carotene. Based on the amount of lipid present, the concentration of vitamin A is much higher in skim milk than in milk fat globules. These observations indicate the likelihood that the vitamin A of milk is disposed in membranes.

It is logical to ascribe the presence of vitamin A in milk to nutritional needs of the newborn mammal. However, the mammary gland and the lactating mammary cell also require this vitamin for proper maintenance and function. While the role of vitamin A at the molecular level in meeting these needs is not known, it may have some generalized function in secretory processes. When epidermal tissue of chick embryo is grown in a medium enriched in vitamin A (retinol), the cells which normally produce keratin are transformed to synthesis and secretion of mucus.[100,288] Lewis[217] has presented evidence of vitamin A, existing mainly as the ester, in membrane material of human and bovine mucus. He concurs with the speculations of Lucy[224] that vitamin A as the alcohol may be important in the secretion process by its facilitation of membrane fusion. Milk represents a useful medium in which to explore this matter. The membranes involved in milk secretion contain vitamin A and pass into the milk. Since the membranous vesicles of the skim milk can be isolated,[292,348] their contents are also worthy of investigation.

H. Lipogenesis in milk and milk as a living system

Milk is often termed "a living tissue" and it is well known for its wide spectrum of enzymatic activities. However, the demonstration[238] that fresh milk can accomplish the net synthesis of triglyceride without benefit of cofactors has opened up additional research possibilities. It is now evident that fresh milk contains glycerol kinase, acyl transferase, stearyl desaturase and the complete system for synthesis of triglyceride by the glycerol-3-phosphate pathway.[187,236,281] Freshly secreted goats milk contains up to 30 μ mol/l of ATP (I. M. Zulak and S. Patton, unpublished). The principal site of this lipogenic activity is the skim milk phase and the incorporation of fatty acids into lipids is localized in a fraction that has since been shown to be a concentrate of membranous vesicles.[281,348] This suggests the possibility that these membranes might be used to study fat droplet formation and membrane biosynthesis. The fact that milk contains membrane fragments provided an opportunity to study their size, a matter which might give insight to origin and structure of membranes. Virtually all of the membrane material in bovine and caprine milks were excluded into the void volume on gel filtration under conditions in which particles of molecular weight < 20 million would have been bound.[291] If membranes of the lactating cell are synthesized from subunits it appears that there is no evidence of these in milk, even though all manner of cell debris occurs therein.

Finally there are the research possibilities offered by the presence of cells in milk. While it is well known that milk from a healthy gland contains bacteria in some numbers, even under the most aseptic conditions of collection, and leucocytes, it was not viewed as a source of mammary epithelial cells. Evidence that these cells occur in some abundance in human milk[56] adds another valuable dimension to the research approach for the mammary gland—one that may have special significance in studies of cell transformation and malignancy. As noted elsewhere (p. 43), cells in milk can be induced to grow in culture.

One of the truly difficult problems in cell and membrane research is to provide samples that are physiologically valid and free of artifacts. Milk provides an approach that overcomes many of the difficulties involved in disintegrating and fractionating tissue.

I. *Biosynthesis of milk lipids in relation to milk technology and food value*

Milk is a product of metabolism and its composition and properties can be specified within the limits of our capacity to understand and manage the metabolism. This has been demonstrated very clearly by the work of Scott and his colleagues,[323,324] wherein the knowledge of rumen function was used to design a feed containing polyunsaturated lipid that would escape hydrogenation in the rumen and lead to substantially unsaturated milk fat.

There are several ways in which lipid metabolism relates in a practical way to milk. We have already alluded to flavor. The levels of various kinds of fatty acids of milk fat (bovine) have characteristic effects on flavor, good or bad depending on circumstances. An excellent treatise by Forss[102] in this series reviews flavor chemistry of lipids including milk and milk products. In addition, a concise review of milk fat flavor potential has been presented by Kinsella *et al.*[193] Another relationship of metabolism is to the nutritive value of milk. Some of the specific factors would concern fat-soluble vitamins (A, D, E and K), cholesterol, essential fatty acid, polyunsaturated fatty acids and calories. The vitamin A potency of milk and milk products involves retinol, its esters and provitamin A (carotene), the latter also representing a color factor. Yet another consideration is the relationship between physical properties of milk and milk products and properties and quantities of milk fat. Whipping of cream, texture of butter are appropriate examples. Physical properties of foods are entwined with considerations of flavor and nutrition as they in turn involve palatability, extent and duration of appetite satisfaction, etc. Clearly lipids are a central concern in such factors.

While the scope of the foregoing subject is large indeed and beyond the needs to treat here, we draw attention, by way of example, to an appropriate contemporary problem. The membrane material in bovine skim milk contains virtually all of the cholesterol and phospholipid therein. Suppression or removal of this material would render skim milk lower in cholesterol, of possible merit in achieving low cholesterol diets, and lower in autoxidizable lipids (phospholipids), which would improve the flavor-keeping quality of skim milk and products made therefrom, e.g. non-fat dry milk, pudding and cake mixes, etc. Recent research at our laboratory has shown that short milking intervals (1 hr) produced depressions in the cholesterol and phospholipid of goat skim milk to as low as one-third initial values.[285] In the experimental results

TABLE 10. *Cholesterol Content (mg) per Serving of Some Common Foods of Animal Origin*[a]

	Cholesterol (mg)		Cholesterol (mg)
Liver (3 1/2 oz serving)	300	Whole milk (8 oz glass)	27
Egg (1 large)	275	Aged cheese (1 oz)	25
Oysters (5 to 8)	200	Ice cream (1/4 pint)	23
Lobster (3 1/2 oz serving)	200	Cottage cheese (1/2 cup)	14
Shrimp (10 small)	125	Butter (1 pat)	12
Veal (3 1/2 oz serving)	90	Gouda cheese (1 oz)	10
Pork (3 1/2 oz serving)	70	Yogurt (1/2 cup)	5
Lamb (3 1/2 oz serving)	70	Skim milk (8 oz glass)	5
Freshwater fish (3 1/2 oz)	70		

[a]Data courtesy of the National Dairy Council.

shown (Fig. 24), the final values (10 hr) are 50% of those at the first hour. Apparently short milking intervals produce a period of reduced sloughing of cell surface, such as of microvilli and vesicles which are known to enter milk.[347] Homer and Virtanen[139] have observed that cholesterol of milk is elevated during the colostral period, during late lactation and during protein-free feeding periods. It appears that additional research might provide milks of lower cholesterol content than those currently available. Actually milk and milk products are relatively modest sources of cholesterol in comparison to other common foods of animal origin (Table 10).

An interesting concept advanced by Reiser and Sidelman[304] is that a high cholesterol intake in early life of the mammal may tend to effect a lifelong suppression of serum cholesterol levels through conditioning to produce less endogenous cholesterol. A related consideration is the recent report that milks contain inhibitors of cholesterol synthesis by rat liver *in vivo* or *in vitro*.[35] Orotic acid appears to be the active inhibiting principle (see Bernstein *et al.*, Addendum).

V. COMPOSITION OF MILK LIPIDS

Having considered background information about general metabolism of the animal and the development and functioning of the mammary tissue, we come to a detailed consideration of the milk lipids, which are products and records of the lactating cell's activities. Milk lipids have simultaneously interested and frustrated investigators. The lipids are readily available, as for example in butter, but are exceptionally complex, both with respect to lipid classes and the component fatty acids. In addition, the latter have been difficult to analyze because of the short-chain fatty acids present and the large number of fatty acids in general. Jenness and Patton[154] in 1959 listed sixteen fatty acids as being in milk lipids, with the possibility of many more. By 1967,[159] the list had grown to approximately 150 and at the present time is over 400.

This extraordinary burst of activity was due to the application of several chromatographic procedures to the separation and identification of milk lipids. James and Martin[153] in 1956 published the first gas–liquid chromatographic (GLC) analysis of milk fatty acids and by 1960 many laboratories were using GLC for routine analysis of these compounds. For example, Jensen et al.[158] reported in 1962 the fatty acid compositions of 106 milk fat samples taken over a period of a year. For comparison, Hansen and Shorland[128] in 1952 analyzed only six samples in a year, using distillation of methyl esters.

Column and thin-layer chromatography (TLC) were also put into use at about the same time as GLC with the latter rapidly coming to the fore because of its speed, ease of use, versatility, resolving power and, probably most important, ease of visualization. TLC has been of enormous value in separating lipid classes, allowing tentative identifications by comparison to knowns, and checking purity. Jensen et al.[161] may well have been the first to separate milk lipid classes with TLC, when in 1961 they used the procedure to obtain diacylglycerols from lipolyzed milk fat.

In 1970 Morrison[245] published a comprehensive review on the composition of milk lipids. He drew attention to the many lipids found in milk fat during the time of intensive research which started about 1958. Since approximately 1967, milk lipids have not received as much attention as in the past, but investigation continues. In this section we present an expansion of the recent review by Jensen.[157] Beyond the material presented in preceding sections, specific effects of environmental, nutritional and genetic factors on the fatty acid composition of milk lipids are not further considered, and in general, only bovine milk lipids are included. Human milk lipids composition has been thoroughly reviewed in a recent book.[111]

TABLE 11. *Composition of Lipids in Whole Bovine Milk*[157]

Lipid	Weight %
Hydrocarbons	tr
Sterol esters	tr
Triacylglycerols	97 – 98
Diacylglycerols	0.28 – 0.59
Monoacylglycerols	0.016 – 0.038
Free fatty acids	0.10 – 0.44
Free sterols	0.22 – 0.41
Phospholipids	0.2 – 1.0

A. *Lipid classes*

1. *Composition*

The composition of bovine whole milk lipids, presented in Table 11, contains no surprises, with the triacylglycerols (TGs) making up the bulk of the material. The partial acylglycerols and free fatty acids are in part remnants of biosynthesis, as they are found in milk that has been extracted immediately after being drawn, before much lipolysis could occur and without any intervening separation treatment other than TLC. The phospholipids and sterols (cholesterol) are obtained primarily from membrane material and the other less polar lipids "accompany" the TGs.

2. *Triacylglycerols*

The composition of milk triacylglycerols (TGs) refers to their structure and ultimately to the identity of individual molecular species. Because there are over 400 fatty acids in an individual sample of milk fat, there could be, based on random distribution, a total of 400^3 or 64×10^6 individual TGs including all positional and enantiomeric isomers, the identification of which would keep generations of biochemical taxonomists busy and happy. A random distribution is here defined as all possible combinations resulting from expansion of the bionomial equation. If we have only two fatty acids, x and y, located at random in the three positions of glycerol then the equation becomes $(x + y)^3$ or $x^3 + 3x^2y + 3xy^2 + y^3$ which when expanded further is:

$$x^3 = xxx,\ 3x^2y = xxy,\ 3yx^2 = yyx,\ y^3 = yyy$$
$$yxx \qquad\qquad xyy$$
$$xyx \qquad\qquad yxy$$

Thus eight TG species are possible including two sets of enantiomers; xxy, yxx and yyx, xyy.

However, a totally random distribution of fatty acids would presume the following conditions: (a) The primary and secondary hydroxyls of sn-3-glycerol phosphate are esterified at the same rates by one or more acyltransferases. (b) All fatty acids are transferred at the same rates regardless of length, degree of unsaturation or the presence of other functional groups in the chain. (c) All fatty acid pools are equally available. In the mammary gland, the rate-controlling enzyme involved could well be blood serum lipoprotein lipase, which hydrolyzes serum TGs in preparation for transport of fatty acids from blood to the gland. (d) The acyltransferase esterifying the sn-1-position of sn-3-glycerol phosphate or sn-2-monoacyl-3-glycerolphosphate behaves the same as the enzyme esterifying the free hydroxyl of sn-1, 2-diacylglycerol. (e) All species of phosphatidic acid are converted to different TGs at the same rate. We either know or can readily assume that none of these conditions apply and therefore a random distribution cannot be expected. Furthermore, the concept of random distribution implies that the sn-1- and 3-hydroxyls of glycerol are identical. We know they are not because the molecule has a chiral center. As we shall discuss later, the structure of milk TGs is asymmetric.

Although milk fat does contain more than 400 fatty acids, Kuksis[202] has pointed out that a more realistic number to deal with is 20, as most of the remainder are there in trace amounts. This number still leaves, however, the possibility of 8000 TGs, but the asymmetry of milk TGs reduces the number further, because all possible enantiomers would not be synthesized. Nevertheless, the several thousand TGs that are undoubtedly in milk fat present intriguing but exasperating problems in identification. Milk TG structure has been reviewed by Jensen and Sampugna,[160] Kuksis and Breckenridge,[203] Morrison,[245] Storry[349] and Kuksis.[202]

(a) *Methods of analysis.* Procedures for separation and structure determination of TGs in general have been described by Litchfield[222] and Kuksis[202] and for milk TGs by Kuksis and Breckenridge[203] and Shehata and de Man.[329] Commonly, chromatographic techniques are used to fractionate the samples and the structure of the TGs in the fractions ascertained by either pancreatic lipase analysis alone or by stereospecific analysis[49] followed by identification of the component fatty acids with GLC. The former identifies the acids in the 1 plus 3 and 2 positions while with the latter the composition of 1, 2 and 3 positions are separately determined. The molecular weight of the TGs is also determined by GLC.

Kuksis and Breckenridge[203] have described an integrated TLC–GLC–lipase analytical system for the analysis of milk TGs which is presented in Fig. 27. The sample was separated into short-, medium- and long-chain fractions by preparative TLC and the molecular distribution and fatty acid composition of each determined by GLC. These fractions were then further separated by argentation TLC into double bond groups and again their molecular weight distribution and fatty acid composition obtained. Preparative GLC was applied to short-chain TGs of uniform molecular weight and degree of unsaturation from the argentation TLC step. Then the fractions were subjected to pancreatic lipase hydrolysis and stereo-specific analysis, the fatty acids, diacylglycerols (DGs) and monoacylglycerols (MGs) from these operations analyzed by GLC and finally the data reconstituted by calculation. A sample of milk TGs obtained by molecular distillation containing mostly TGs made up of two medium- or long-chain fatty acids associated with one short-chain fatty acid was also subjected to stereospecific analysis. Later Kuksis et al.[204] using GLC with polyester columns were able to resolve butyryl, caproyl and caprylyl TGs with identical numbers of acyl carbons and double bonds. It is obvious that these procedures will produce a forbiddingly large number of samples.

Nutter and Privett[258] combined liquid–liquid chromatography and argentation TLC for the analysis of milk TG structure. Positional isomers (pancreatic lipase) were not determined because the authors doubted that the lipase would randomly hydrolyze TGs containing short-chain acids.

Shehata et al.[331,332] also integrated several procedures for milk TG analysis, separating the fat into seventeen major fractions by silicic acid column chromatography which were then fractionated by argentation-TLC. The TGs and fatty acids in all samples were determined by GLC.

A paper[211] describing the separation of non-polar lipids by high-speed liquid chromatography has recently appeared. Monopalmitin, palmitic acid, 1,3-dipalmitin, cholesterol and tripalmitin were separated on a column of polystyrene gel with aqueous acetone in 30 min. The materials were quantitated with a moving wire flame ionization detector. Although this method offers the advantage of speed, it has apparently not been applied to the separation of milk TGs and indeed, this application would probably require different columns, eluting solvents and detection procedures.

Murata and Takahashi[251] have applied GLC-mass spectrometry to the analysis of milk TGs and several other fats. The samples were first separated on the basis of molecular weight (carbon number) by GLC and the component acids identified by mass spectrometry. The number of double bonds per molecular weight in each carbon number unit starting with 50 was also determined, but carbon numbers less than 46 were not reported for milk fat, although they were given for coconut oil. The major advantages of the technique are speed and the small amount of sample required.

At present, two procedures are employed to isolate and identify the acids in the various positions of TGs. These are lipolysis with pancreatic lipase and stereospecific analyses.[222] It is well known that pancreatic lipase is almost completely specific for the primary esters of TGs usually hydrolyzing the acids esterified at these positions in equimolar quantities regardless of chain length.[51,156] It was earlier believed that pancreatic lipase analysis would give misleading results because of presumed preferential hydrolysis of the short-chain acids. The problem was found to be preferential lipolysis of TGs containing short-chain acids. Sampugna et al.[316] observed the follow-

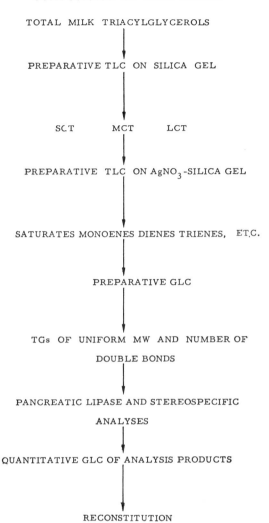

FIG. 27. Flow sheet of the integrated thin-layer chromatography (TLC)–gas–liquid chromatography (GLC)–lipase system used by Kuksis and Breckenridge[203] to determine the structure of milk triglycerides.

ing decreasing rates of hydrolysis by pancreatic lipase: PBB > PPB > PBP > P-B where P and B were 16:0 and 4:0 in the synthetic racemic glycerides. Both P and B were released from PBB in equimolar quantities. These findings indicate that individual milk TG species or groups thereof would be digested representatively by pancreatic lipase.

Stereospecific analysis identifies the fatty acids located in the sn-1, 2 and 3 positions of TGs.[50] DGs are generated by pancreatic lipolysis or by reaction with methyl magnesium bromide, converted to phenyl phosphatides then exposed to phospholipase 2 (A_2)[51] which hydrolyzes the sn-3-phosphatide and not the sn-1 species. Stereospecific analysis does not determine the arrangement of fatty acids into TGs. Brockerhoff[50] employed the Grignard reagent because in some instances, pancreatic lipase was not

TABLE 12. *Distribution of the Individual Fatty Acids in Bovine Milk Triacylglycerols*[290]

Fatty acid	sn-position (mole %)		
	1	2	3
4:0	9.8	5.6	84.6
6:0	16.3	25.8	58.0
8:0	17.2	42.1	40.7
10:0	20.7	49.7	29.6
12:0	24.6	47.5	28.0
14:0	27.6	53.8	18.6
16:0	45.5	41.7	12.8
16:1	48.5	35.6	15.9
18:0	58.2	25.9	16.0
18:1	41.8	27.9	30.3
18:2	36.7	77.9	−14.6

producing DGs which were representative of the original TGs. Kuksis et al.[204] have shown that both deacylation techniques produced identical results when fractions of milk fat were analyzed, the length of pancreatic lipolysis was 4 min and diethyl ether was added to the digestion mixture. In short, under these circumstances, pancreatic lipolysis will result in DGs representative of the original TGs which can then be employed in stereospecific analysis.

(b) *Structure*. The most striking feature of milk TG structure is the asymmetry; the almost exclusive location of 4:0, 6:0 and 8:0 in the sn-3 position with longer chain acids in the other two positions of the TGs. This was first determined by Pitas et al.[290] and by Breckenridge and Kuksis[42] and has since been extensively verified. Pitas et al.[290] made the determination on unfractionated milk fat and the results are presented in Table 12. It can be noted that enantiomeric TGs were obviously present as the compositions of positions sn-1 and 3 were markedly dissimilar.

Breach et al.[41] calculated the randomness of association of different fatty acids in milk TGs from various animals and found that it was more or less non-random in all species. They postulated that the intermolecular specificity could be explained by positional specificity of fatty acids on the glycerol molecule.

The results of exhaustive structural analyses by Kuksis and colleagues have been determined in reviews[202,203] to which the reader is referred. Kuksis et al.[204] summarized their findings as follows: There are three basic types of milk TGs. The first type has acyl carbons of 48-54 composed of long-chain 1,2-DGs acylated by 18:0, 18:1 and 18:2. With type 2 the carbon numbers are 36–46 and the sn-3 position acids are 4:0, 6:0 and 8:0. These TGs are enantiomers. In type 3, the carbon numbers are 26–34, the 1,2-DGs contain medium-chain acids and the 3-position acids are short and medium chain. Those TGs in type 3 that have short-chain acids in the sn-3 position or medium-chain acids in sn-3 that are different from those in sn-1 are also enantiomers.

Shehata et al.[332] have somewhat bravely named individual milk TGs from data based on their argentation TLC and molecular weight separations. Some of their data are presented in Table 13. These data combined with the information obtained by Murata and Takahashi[251] with GLC-mass spectrometry and the findings of Kuksis

TABLE 13. *Major Individual Triacylglycerols in Two Bovine Milk Fat Fractions*[332]

TG type	Carbon number species	Mole %	Major individual TGs
SMS[a]	50	24.3	16, 18:1, 16[b] 18, 18:1, 14
SSM	50	30.8	18:1, 18, 14 18:1, 16, 16

[a]SMS is saturate–monoene–saturate.
[b]Acids are not arranged positionally.

above allow us to make some reasonably reliable identifications. If we consider the two major TGs in carbon number 50, 14-18-18 and 16-16-18 then refer to the double bond and the TG types, SSM or SMS in Table 13 and to data in Table 14, 14-18-18 could be *rac* 14:0-18:0-18:1, *rac* 14:0-18:1-18:0, or *rac* 18:0-14:0-18:1. Since Breckenridge and Kuksis[43] found more 14:0 in *sn*-2 than in *sn*-1 and reverse concentrations of 18:0 in these positions for long-chain TGs, we can assume that one of the TGs was *sn*-1-18:0-14:0-18:1. Readers may wish to similarly amuse themselves.

The important point to remember concerning milk TG structure is the asymmetry; the *sn*-3 location of the short-chain fatty acids. Physiologically, milk fat will be uniquely metabolized. Those TGs with short-chain fatty acids will be digested more rapidly as molecules than the long-chain TGs by pancreatic lipase and the short-chain acids transported via the portal vein to the liver where they will be oxidized. The reconstituted TGs emerging into the chyle from the intestinal wall will not contain the short-chain acids and some of the medium-chain acids will also be missing.

3. Other acylglycerols

If some of the diacylglycerols (DGs) in freshly drawn milk are involved in biosynthesis it is possible that they are enantiomeric, and probably the *sn*-1,2 isomer. If so, the constituent fatty acids would be long chain (see the analysis of mammary tissue lipids by Patton and McCarthy[279]). The configuration could be determined by stereospecific analysis,[49] but it would be difficult to accumulate enough material for

TABLE 14. *Major Individual Triacylglycerols in a Milk Fat Fraction as Determined by GLC-Mass Spectrometry*[251]

Carbon number	TG species	Mole %	Molecular weight	Mole %	Number of double bonds
50	14-16-20[a]	3	830	14	2[b]
	14-18-18	44	832	32	1
	16-16-18	53	834	54	0

[a]Double bonds disregarded.
[b]Total number of double bond per molecular weight.

analysis. Boudreau and de Man[38] reported DG contents of 4.4–6.6% in milk fat; these are very high and probably resulted from the isolation technique used. Unless freshly drawn milk is heated or extracted immediately to inactivate the lipase, lipolysis commences and is accelerated by pipeline milking. Processed milk always contains partial acylglycerols and free fatty acids partially as a result of lipolysis, but the quantities are small.[161,354] Chromatographic separation of lipids on basic alumina also leads to high diglyceride values.

Timmen and Dimick[354] characterized the major hydroxy compounds in milk lipids by first isolating the compounds as their pyruvic ester-2,6-dinitrophenylhydrazones. Concentrations as weight percent of the compounds from bovine herd milk lipids were: 1,2-DGs 1.43, hydroxyacylglycerols 0.61 and sterols 0.35. Lipolysis tripled the DG content. The usual milk fatty acids were observed, except that the DGs lacked 4:0 and 6:0 again indicating that these lipids were in part intermediates in milk lipid biosynthesis. If so, then these DGs would be the *sn*-1,2-isomers. With the large hydrazone group attached to the hydroxyl the derivatives should appreciably rotate polarized light and would therefore be detectable with a polarimeter.

Diol lipids are not listed, but might be present. These compounds, discussed in a recent review by Bergelson,[24] have been detected in several mammalian tissues and in seeds. If in milk lipids, diol lipids would be masked by TGs.

Alkyl and alk-1-enyl ether diacylglycerols are also found in milk lipids.[245] Parks et al.[264] detected 0.2 μM of bound aldehyde per g of butterfat and identified n-9 through 18 and br-11, 13, 15, 16 and 17 aldehydes. The aldehydes were derived from the alk-1-enyl ether-diacylglycerols. Glyceryl ethers, -alkyl ether diacylglycerols were found in milk fat at a level of 0.10% and the 16:0, 18:0 and 18:1 acyl chains determined.[125]

4. *Phospholipids*

The phospholipid composition of milk is tabulated in Table 15.[157] There has been only one new addition to the list since mid-1968, gangliosides,[145,167,171] but several of the components have been more thoroughly analyzed as will be discussed later.

TABLE 15. *Phospholipid Composition of Bovine Milk*[157]

Phospholipid	M%
Phosphatidyl choline	34.5
Phosphatidyl ethanolamine	31.8
Phosphatidyl serine	3.1
Phosphatidyl inositol	4.7
Sphingomyelin	25.2
Lysophosphatidyl choline	tr
Lysophosphatidyl ethanolamine	tr
Total choline phospholipids	59.7
Plasmalogens	3
Diphosphatidyl glycerol	tr
Ceramides	tr
Cerebrosides	tr
Gangliosides[a]	tr

[a]References 145, 167 and 171.

Diphosphatidyl glycerol (cardiolipin) was found in lactating mammary tissue at levels 200-300 times the amount found in milk.[274] The authors attributed this difference to selectivity during milk secretion.

Lysophosphatides are presumably always present, but whether or not these are artifacts of isolation or fragments of biosynthesis is unknown. A determination of the structure of these compounds, e.g., *sn*-1-or *sn*-2-monoacyl, should provide useful information.

Phosphatidyl serine has been analyzed by Boatman *et al.*[33] who found contents of 2.4-3.4%, as percentage of total lipid P. In the same paper, 37.6-40.9% quantities of phosphatidyl ethanolamine were noted as well as ceramide mono- and dihexosides (cerebrosides).

Cerebrosides were earlier reported by, among others, Nutter and Privett[257] and have been recently analyzed more completely by Kayser and Patton[166] who observed partitioning of the compounds between milk fat globules and the serum portion of milk in a manner paralleling the phospholipids. They also identified glucosyl and lactosyl ceramides. Morrison and Hay[248] have published comprehensive data on the composition of both these compounds.

Milk sphingomyelin has been investigated by Fujino and Fujishima[110] and Morrison and Hay,[248] all of whom identified the fatty acids and sphingosine bases present. These data will be presented subsequently.

Huang[145] found relatively high concentrations of gangliosides in buttermilk; 10-20 mg per g of total lipid as compared to 0.5 mg in brain lipids. Buttermilk is the watery fluid which separates from butter when the latter is churned from cream and should not be confused with the cultured product, which is made from skim milk by addition of a lactic culture. The ganglioside fraction, obtained by silica gel column chromatography, was divided into five components by TLC. Two of these were identified: one as neuraminosyl (2 → 8) neuraminosyl (2 → 3) lactosyl ceramide (50%) and the other as neuraminosyl (2 → 3) lactosyl ceramide (20%). The other three compounds were not characterized because of the small quantities available. Data on the fatty acids and sphingosine bases will be given later.

There are many other phospholipids which have been found in both microorganisms[6] and plants[112] that might be expected to appear in milk, but whose presence has not been reported. Among these are phosphonolipids, as several have been identified in rumen protozoa.[366]

5. Sterols

These compounds are found in the unsaponifiable fraction of milk lipids and are mostly cholesterol with some lanosterol. Recently, Brewington *et al.*[46] confirmed the presence of the latter sterol and identified two new constituents, dihydrolanosterol and β-sitosterol. Some of the many sterol precursors of cholesterol may also be present in trace amounts, but have not been isolated and identified. Keenan and Patton[178] have reported on the cholesterol esters of milk lipids. These represent about one-tenth of the sterol content of milk.

Reliable data on the cholesterol content of dairy products, lacking in the past, have recently become available.[206] The amount in whole milk fat was 13.49 ± 1.01 mg per 100 g milk which contained 3.47 ± 0.74 g of fat. Data were obtained from 27 kinds of products and from these an equation was derived for estimating the cholesterol content of dairy products with fat contents greater than whole milk. The equation is: $Y = 6.34 + 2.83\ X$, where $Y =$ mg cholesterol per 100 g of food and $X =$ mg fat per 100 g of food. It is obvious that more fat is accompanied by more cholesterol, e.g., cheddar cheese contained 102 mg per 100 g, an approximate 8-fold concentration over whole milk. As an aid for the worried dieter, creamed cottage cheese contained 14 mg per g, and the low fat variety 6 mg, while skim milk had 2 mg per 100 g. For further discussion of cholesterol, see Section IV.

6. *Hydrocarbons*

Milk lipids contain small quantities of various hydrocarbons: carotenoids, squalene, etc.[157,245] Ristow and Warner[308] identified the C-14 to C-35 n-alkanes and some branched monolefins, but solely on the basis of GLC retention times. Flanagan and Ferretti[101] using GLC-mass spectrometry found 39 aliphatic hydrocarbons in the unsaponifiable fraction of anhydrous milk fat. The compounds were the C-14 to C-27 and C-29 to C-31 straight chain paraffins, their monolefin analogs and the C-25 to C-29 branched alkanes. Phytene was identified for the first time in milk fat and polychlorinated biphenyls (PCBs) were also present. The total hydrocarbons amounted to 30 ppm of the milk fat. The PCBs were undoubtedly adventitious interlopers as they have been widely used in paints, plastics, etc.

7. *Lipoproteins*

As pointed out elsewhere[54] and in preceding sections the bulk of the lipoprotein of milk is membrane, membrane around milk fat globules and as vesicles and fragments in the skim milk. Membrane is found in milk at a concentration of about 0.1% and appears to be mainly plasma membrane derived from the lactating cell.

The results of detailed analyses of the lipid composition of fat globule membranes from bovine milk have been published by Bracco et al.,[39] Peereboom[287] and Prentice.[299] Bracco *et al.* found the high melting TGs and other lipids observed by previous investigators.[54] Approximately 62% TGs were present, much less than in the parent milk lipid. Among the hydrocarbons isolated, squalene was positively identified with indications by GLC of odd and even alkanes, alkenes and polyunsaturated compounds between C-31 and C-38. In addition to cholesterol, 7-dehydrocholesterol was detected;

TABLE 16. *Composition of the Lipids from the Milk Fat Globule Membrane*[39,157]

Lipid component	Percent of membrane lipids
Carotenoids	0.45
Squalene	0.61
Cholesterol esters	0.79
Triacylglycerols	53.4
Free fatty acids	6.3[a]
Cholesterol	5.2
Diacylglycerols	8.1
Monoacylglycerols	4.7
Phospholipids	20.4

[a] Contained some TGs.

other hydrocarbons tentatively identified were carotenoids and tocopherols. Phospholipid classes were noted in relative quantities not greatly different from those in Table 15. Berlin et al.[25] analyzed microsome (membrane) material from the skim milk phase and found it to be 87% lipid of which 52% was phospholipid and 35% neutral lipid.

Summarized data on milk fat globule membrane lipids can be seen in Table 16. The free fatty acid and partial acylglycerol contents are probably too high. The former fraction contained some TGs.[54] Bracco et al.[39] found lower quantities of all these lipid classes. These investigators determined the positional distribution of the component fatty acids within the membrane TGs finding relatively larger quantities of 12:0, 14:0, 16:0 and 18:0 in position 2, than in unfractionated milk TGs.

B. Composition of lipid classes

1. Determination of fatty acids

GLC is still the method of choice for the routine separation and tentative identification of common milk fatty acids, as well as the resolution of the less abundant and less common acids. Although several hundred fatty acids are listed here and elsewhere[157,159,245] as being present in milk, we remind the reader that not all of these were rigorously identified. Some of the pitfalls in qualitative and quantitative GLC of milk fatty acids are discussed by Jensen et al.[159] and of fatty acids in general by Ackman.[1] Dickes and Nicholas[79] have recently published a paper reviewing the applications of GLC to the analysis of milk and dairy products. This paper is particularly helpful as the authors discuss esterification methods, GLC columns, etc.

As always in the analysis of milk fat, the short-chain fatty acids cause problems. The major difficulty has not been the GLC separation of these acids, but in transferring them from the esterification mixture to the GLC instrument without loss of the volatile esters. The best procedure we have found is a slight modification of the method developed by Christopherson and Glass[66] which uses sodium methoxide for transesterification. This technique can be employed with other fats, but not with those containing appreciable amounts of free fatty acids where HCl-methanol is required. The procedure is described in detail as follows:

(a) To a vessel, usually a small pear-shaped flask containing 2 drops (about 50 mg) of fat from which the extracting solvent has been evaporated, add 5 ml of 2N sodium methoxide. Stopper, swirl and allow to stand at room temperature for about 15 min.

(b) Transfer esterification mixture to an 8% Babcock milk fat test bottle, rinse the flask with 1 ml of petroleum ether (30–60) and transfer the rinse to the Babcock bottle. Add H_2O until the mixture is at the top of the graduated neck and centrifuge the bottle at 800–1000 rpm for a few minutes. For the uninitiated, a Babcock test bottle has a long graduated neck and is available at low cost from most laboratory supply firms.

(c) Withdraw the desired amount of petroleum ether–methyl ester solution, which is now at the top of the graduated neck, with a micro-syringe and inject directly into the GLC instrument.

Shehata et al.[330] have described a somewhat similar procedure in which the esterification mixture can be injected directly into the GLC instrument from the reaction vial.

In order to analyze milk fat, the investigator must first, in the words of Gurr and James,[123] "catch his lipid". The methods and problems involved have been discussed by Morrison.[245] Most of the lipids, with the exception of very polar phospholipids, can be extracted by the Roese–Gottleib method,[10] but a more satisfactory procedure is the modified Folch technique used by Timmen and Dimick.[354] Because the quantities of lipids other than TGs in milk are relatively low, spray dried buttermilk, in which phospholipids are concentrated about 25-fold,[245] is often used as a source of these compounds, with the assumption that the processing does not markedly alter the composition. For further information on the isolation, analysis and identification of lipids, we refer the reader to the cited references and the manual by Kates.[163]

2. *Fatty acids in general*

A list of 142 fatty acids then believed to be in milk lipids was compiled by Jensen et al.[159] in 1967. The quantities in the list (Table 17) are representatives of milk lipids, but quantities in individual samples may vary since the amounts were taken from many references. To supplement the table, all the odd chain acids between 2:0–28:0 were found; all odd chain acids were in the monoenes except 11:1, with positional and geometric isomers; the dienes were even chain with some conjugated geometric isomers; the polyenes were all even with some conjugated *trans* isomers; the monobranched acids did not contain 10:0 but did have both iso and anteiso and the multibranched acids were both odd and even with three to five methyl branches.

Hay and Morrison[133] studied the monoenoic positional and geometric isomers in bovine milk fat finding *cis* Δ 5 – 8, 14:1; *cis* Δ 5 – 12, 16:1; *trans* Δ 5 – 14, 16:1; *cis* Δ 6 – 12, 17:1; *cis* Δ 8 – 11, 18:1 and *trans* Δ 6 – 16, 18:1. The Δ 9 isomers and several of the positional isomers of 18:1 had been detected earlier. See Table 18 for these data. The work of Hay and Morrison added 37 additional acids to the list in Table 17.

Strocchi and Holman,[350] with the aid of argentation-TLC and GLC-mass spectrometry, identified more monoenoic acids as follows: *trans* 17:1, 19:1, 20:1, 21:1, 22:1, 23:1 and 24:1. Notably missing was 11:1, either *cis* or *trans*. Presumably the terminal

TABLE 17. *Fatty Acid Composition of Milk Lipids*, circa 1967[a]

Acids[b]	Quantity (wt %)
2:0 – 28:0	63.0
10:1 – 26:1	31.0
14:2 – 26:2	2.3
18:3, 20:3, 20:4, 22:3, 22.4, 22:5, 22:6	0.9
Monobranched – 9:0 – 26:0	1.4
Multibranched – 16:0 – 28:0	0.8
Keto – 10:0 – 18:0, 18:1	tr
Hydroxyl – 10:0 – 16:0	tr
Cyclic – 17:0	tr

[a]Adapted from ref. 159.
[b]Positional and geometric isomers not designated. See text.

TABLE 18. *Positional and Geometric Isomers of Bovine Milk Lipid Monoenoic Fatty Acids*[a] (wt %)

Position of double bond	cis isomers				trans isomers	
	14:1	16:1	17:1	18:1	16:1	18:1
5	1.0	tr			2.2	
6	0.8	1.3	3.4		7.8	1.0
7	0.9	5.6	2.1		6.7	0.8
8	0.6	tr	20.1	1.7	5.0	3.2
9	96.6	88.7	71.3	95.8	32.8	10.2
10		tr	tr	tr	1.7	10.5
11		2.6	2.9	2.5	10.6	35.7
12		tr	tr		12.9	4.1
13					10.6	10.5
14						9.0
15						6.8
16						7.5

[a] Adapted from ref. 248.

methyl group of a saturated fatty acid must be three or more carbons beyond C-9 before desaturation can occur during biosynthesis in the mammary gland. We have included all the data of Strocchi and Holman (Tables 19 and 20) because the identifications were obtained by unequivocal means, they confirm many previously tentative

TABLE 19. *Fatty Acid Composition of Butter Oil as Determined by GLC-Mass Spectrometry* (wt %) *of total methyl esters*[a]

Methyl ester carbons	Saturates	Monoenes		Branched		
		cis	trans	iso	anteiso	other
4	3.25					
6	2.32					
8	1.85					
10	4.02					
11	0.16					
12	4.15	0.03				
13	0.03			0.01	tr	
14	11.05	0.47		0.08		
15	0.95	0.08		0.23	0.42	
16	26.15	1.25	0.03	0.32		
17	0.70	0.32	0.01	0.33	0.40	DDL pristanate, 0.01
18	9.60	0.40	5.34	0.15		
19	0.11	0.10	0.01	0.06	0.09	DDD pristanate, 0.01
20	0.19	0.15	0.01	0.04		DDL, DDD phytanates, 0.04
21	0.06	0.03	tr	tr	0.01	
22	0.10	0.02	tr	tr		
23	0.07	0.01	0.01			
24	0.06	0.02	0.01			
25	0.01					
26	0.04					

[a] Adapted from ref. 350.

TABLE 20. *Fatty Acid Composition of Butter Oil as Determined by GLC-Mass Spectrometry (a continuation of Table 19)*[a]

Methyl ester carbons	Dienes	Trienes	Tetraenes	Pentaenes
		wt % of total methyl esters		
18				
Positional	0.14	0.02		
isomers	2.30	0.60		
Conjugated				
cis, trans	0.70	di-0.03		
trans, trans	0.05	tri-0.01		
20				
Positional	0.03	0.01	0.10	
isomers	tr	0.13	0.02	
		0.02		
22				
Positional	0.04	0.06		0.02
isomers	tr	0.02		0.02
24				
Positional	tr	0.01		
isomers		0.03		
		0.02		

[a]Adapted from ref. 350.

identifications and are quantitative. Strocchi and Holman did not identify the positional isomers of the unsaturates, but found two or three peaks for most of the carbon numbers.

Yet to be completely identified are the large number of isomers that could result from positional and geometrical isomerization of *cis, cis*-9, 12 – 18:2. The same situation applies to 18:3 and the other polyunsaturates. A few conjugated isomers of both acids have been found.[159] Van der Wel and de Jong[362] have identified several *cis, trans* or *trans, cis* and *trans, trans* 18:2 positional isomers other than the 9,12 and the identity of these are presented in Table 21.

TABLE 21. *Location of Double Bonds in Unconjugated* 18:2 *Isomers of Milk Lipids*[a]

cis, cis	cis, trans or trans, cis	trans, trans
11, 15	11, 16 and/or 11, 15	12, 16
10, 15	10, 16 and/or 10, 15	11, 16 and/or 11, 15
9, 15	9, 15 and/or 9, 16	10, 16 and/or 10, 15
8, 15 and/or 8, 12	8, 16 and/or 8, 15	9, 16 and/or 9, 15
7, 15 and/or 7, 12	and/or 8, 12	and/or 9, 13
6, 15 and/or 6, 12		

[a]Adapted from refs. 245 and 362.

Strocchi and Holman[350] noted, but did not further characterize, two or more positional isomers of 18:2, 18:3, 20:2, 20:3, 20:4, 22:2, 22:3, 22:4, 22:5, and 24:3. Also detected were conjugated isomers of 18:2 and 18:3.

Hansen[127] isolated and identified 4,8,12–trimethyltridecanoic acid from milk fat. The acid was the DD disastereoisomer and phytol was believed to be the precursor. Earlier, Ackman and Hansen[2] examined three butterfat samples for phytanic and pristanic acids by an improved GLC method, finding that two contained about twice as much DDD as LDD isomer while the third had approximately equal quantities of both. Egge et al.[89] found at least 50 branched chain fatty acids in human milk fat by identification with GLC-mass spectrometry following hydrogenation and enrichment of the acids by urea fractionation (Table 22). They postulated that many of

TABLE 22. *Branched Chain Fatty Acids of Human Milk Lipids as Determined by GLC-Mass Spectrometry*[a]

n-Chain length	Location of methyl group
10:0	3-5, 7-9[b]
11:0	3-5, 10
12:0	2-8, 10, 11; 3, 7, 11 tri-[c]
13:0	4, 5, 10, 12; 4, 8, 12 tri-
14:0	2, 4-8, 12, 13
15:0	2, 4, 13, 14; 5, 9, 13 tri- 2, 6, 10, 14 tetra-
16:0	7, 8, 12, 14, 15; 3, 7, 11, 15 tetra-
17:0	5, 9, 10, 11, 12, 16;
18:0	10, 11

[a]Adapted from ref. 89
[b]Signifies that monobranched acids with methyl groups on the 3, 4, 5, 7, 8, and 9 carbons were identified.
[c]Signifies three methyl groups, one each at the 3, 7 and 11 carbons.

these were of bacterial origin produced in and absorbed from the intestinal tract. We can assume that application of similar procedures would identify as many or more branched chain acids in bovine milk fat as indicated by Iverson.[151]

With GLC-mass spectrometry, Ryhage[314] identified in milk lipids: 15:0 br acids with the methyl group on the 8, 9, 10, 11, 12 or 14 carbon; iso 12:0, iso 13:0, anteiso 13:0, iso 14:0, iso 16:0 and anteiso 19:0. Iverson[151] concentrated the branched chain acids from milk lipids by urea complexing then tentatively identified the following acids with programmed temperature GLC: all of the odd and even numbered 12:0–26:0 monobranched acids; 16:0, 17:0, 18:0, 16:0 and 28:0 acids with three methyl groups; 19:0–28:0 containing four methyl groups and a 28:0 acid with five groups. Strocchi and Holman[350] confirmed the presence of 2,6,10,14 tetramethylhexadecanoate and DDD and DDL phytanates in bovine milk lipids. Others identified were: 13:0 anteiso, 19:0 iso and anteiso and 21:0 iso and anteiso which were not listed in the compilation of Jensen et al.[159] Monomethylbranched isomers of 15:0 and 17:0 other than iso and anteiso were absent, although several of both were observed in human milk lipids by Egge et al.[89] and in bovine milk by Ryhage.[314]

Ackman et al.[3] analyzed C-15 and C-17 enriched fractions of milk fat with high resolution open-tubular GLC, finding that only even-numbered carbons of the acyl chains bore the methyl branch. In the C-15 fraction, methyl branching occurred at the 4, 6, 8 and 10 carbons and in the C-17, at the 4, 6, 8, 10 and 12 carbons. Most of the iso acids had been removed by prior purification. Ackman et al.[3] suggested that the difficulty of interpreting mass spectra from complex mixtures may have lead to assumptions concerning the existence of monomethyl branches and odd carbon fatty acids.[89] Conversely, several of these acids were identified by Strocci and Holman[350] who analyzed a fraction, obtained by TLC, with GLC-mass spectrometry, containing only n- and monomethyl branched fatty acids. Some of these differences may have been caused by the uniqueness of the individual milk fat samples.

Milk fat contains both keto (oxo) and hydroxy fatty acids and earlier identifications are discussed in refs. 159 and 245. In a recent and careful study, Weihrauch et al.[370] isolated 60 oxo acids from milk fat and positively and tentatively identified 47 with the aid of mass spectrometry. These data are in Table 23. About 85% (wt) of the oxo-acids were stearates, mostly the 13-isomer, and 20% were palmitates, largely the 11-isomer. Of the unsaturated oxo-acids, the 9-oxo-Δ-12 and 13-oxo-Δ-9 were the predominant species. Other unsaturated oxo acids not listed in Table 23, but the presence of which were indicated, were: 15:1, 16:2, 17:1, 17:2, 17:3, 18:2, 18:3, 19:1, 19:2 and 20:1.

Hydroxy acids, 10:0–16:0, with the functional group in the 4 and 5 positions have been found in milk fat, as well as 12:1 Δ 6, 4-OH, and 12:1 Δ 9, 5-OH.[85,159] These isomers convert readily to lactones, some of which are flavor compounds. Schwartz,[322] in a discussion of methods for the isolation of non-lactonegenic hydroxy fatty acids

TABLE 23. n-Oxo Fatty Acids in Milk Fat[a]

Carbon number	Position of carbonyl
10:0	5
12:0	4, 5, 7
14:0	5, 6, 7, 9
15:0	4, 5
16:0	4–9, 11
17:0	8
18:0	5, 8–11, 13, 16
19:0	11
20:0	9, 11, 15
22:0	11–15
24:0	14, 15

	Position of carbonyl and double bond
14:1	5 (Δ9), 5 (Δ 10), 9 (Δ 5)
16:1	7 (Δ 10), 11 (Δ 7), 11 (Δ 9)
18:1	9 (Δ12), 9 (Δ13), 9 (Δ15), 13 (Δ7), 13 (Δ9)

[a]Reference 370.

(OH group on carbons other than 4 or 5), mentioned that there were at least 60 acids in this fraction. In a discussion of milk hydroxy acids, we must not forget those in sphingolipids. These 2-hydroxy acids are listed in Table 33.

In the same presentation mentioned above, Schwartz[322] also noted the detection of about 70 glycerol-1-alkyl ethers in milk fat. Saturated ethers, both odd and even from C-10 through C-18, were found with traces of ethers up to C-25 present. Fifty-five unsaturated ethers were separated but only the Δ-9, Δ-9,12 and Δ-9,12,15 compounds were tentatively identified. In addition, Schwartz isolated over 50 bound aldehydes probably derived from the glycerol-1-alkenyl ethers (phosphorus free).

Two cyclic acids have been isolated from milk fat and characterized; cyclohexylundecanoic acid from both bovine[159] and human milk[89] and cyclohexylnonanoic acid from the latter.

One of the questions that arose during the preparation of this review is, why have not many more fatty acids been found in bovine milk fat? When the large range of fatty acids other than those already found in milk fat and known to be in plant[337] and rumen lipids[137,366] is considered, it is obvious that many more acids than those discussed herein could be present. Where, for example, are the cyclopropane acids? They could be hydrogenated to methyl branched and straight chain acids during passage through the rumen.[65] Also, some of the acid-catalyzed esterification and transesterification procedures may completely destroy or alter cyclopropane acids. Anhydrous methanolic HCl apparently may be used without alteration of the cyclopropane acids as can methanolic boron trichloride.[47] As a stimulus for the search, two cyclopropane acids have been recently found in sheep rumen tissue lipids[34] where they were esterified to the *sn*-1 position of phosphatidylethanolamine. Unexpectedly the acids were identified as 2,3methylene hexadecanoic and octadecanoic and not the anticipated 11,12methylene octadecanoic acid (lactobacillic) which occurs in microorganisms.

Cyclopropane acids, which are certainly consumed by the cow, in among other feeds cottonseed oil cake, may be hydrogenated in the rumen.[65] However, cows fed cottonseed oil, yielded high melting milk fat, which was the result of accumulation of saturated fatty acids and a decrease in oleic acid content. The major cyclopropene acid is sterculic, which is a potent inhibitor of fatty acid desaturase enzymes. It seems likely that the effect of cottonseed oil fed to cows discussed above might be caused by the inhibitory effect of sterculic acid on desaturase enzymes. It follows that the acid may not be hydrogenated in the rumen. This could be easily tested *in vitro*. Sterculic acid administered intravenously to cows causes an increase in the stearic acid content of the milk fat during treatment.[26]

If an investigator uses appropriate methods of concentration, such as urea inclusion, argentation-TLC, GLC-mass spectrometry, etc., it seems possible that most of the many fatty acids found in plant lipids could be detected in milk if a worker is sufficiently motivated to do so. One deterrent to such an endeavor is the very low concentration at which many of these acids may occur in milk fat.

3. *Protected milk*

Bovine milk fat contains relatively low concentrations, about 2%, of polyunsaturated fatty acids as a result of biohydrogenation of dietary lipids in the rumen. Australian investigators found that a polyunsaturated oil encapsulated in sodium caseinate by spray drying followed by a denaturation treatment with formaldehyde to prevent proteolysis of the protein in the rumen, was protected against ruminal hydrogenation.[323] For example, the 18:2 content of milk fat from a cow fed protected particles of safflower oil was 35.2% as compared to 2.0% for the control animal. Protected oils are hydrolyzed in the abomasum and the fatty acids absorbed in the small intestine, thereby avoiding hydrogenation.[324] Results of feeding protected corn and peanut oils to cows, on the fatty acid composition of milk fat, are presented in Table 24. Note that the 14:0, 16:0 and 18:0 contents are reduced while the amounts of 18:2 were increased about five-fold. Similar increases were observed in plasma and depot fats. Investigators at the USDA[32,293] confirmed the findings of the Australian workers; also noting that the 18:2 content of cow's milk fat could be increased from 3% to 35% by feeding protected safflower oil. Thus, it is possible if proved necessary, to biologically increase the polyunsaturated fatty acid content of milk fat. Individuals with Type II hyperlipoproteinemia,[108] who are advised to increase dietary polyunsaturated acids and decrease the saturates in order to reduce plasma cholesterol, would benefit by the availability of "protected" milk, but at the present time it is much more economical for them to drink skim milk and obtain their polyunsaturated fatty acids from the proper margarines, salad oils, etc.

Worth noting are the further efforts of the Australian scientists,[254] who fed diets composed of protected milk, cheese, butter and cream prepared from the milk, and beef and drippings from cows fed the protected oil to six human volunteers. Plasma cholesterol contents were reduced by 10% in five of six subjects. However, the cholesterol contents of the control diet obtained from cattle fed normal rations and test diets were quite similar, ranging from 412mg to 592mg per day. We should mention that the type II hyperlipoproteinemia diet calls for a cholesterol intake of 300 mg per day[108] and that the fat from protected milk will probably not have the tocopherol content of an equivalent vegetable oil. Research on the polyunsaturated milks has not yet made clear the levels of short-chain acids ($<C_{14}$) in the milk fat.

TABLE 24. *The Effects of Feeding Protected Corn and Peanut Composition of Cow's Milk[a] Oils on the Fatty Acid*

Fatty acids	Fatty acid composition of milk lipids, wt %		
	Corn oil	Peanut oil	Control
14:0	7.9	9.7	11.9
16:0	20.5	22:1	31.1
18:0	9.8	11.0	13.5
18:1	28.8	25.3	29.5
18:2	20.1	20.5	4.2
18:3	1.8	2.9	2.7
Others	11.1	8.5	7.1

[a]Oils entrapped in formaldehyde treated casein.
Adapted from ref. 324.

4. Phospholipids

Some of the earlier data tabulated by Morrison[245] on the fatty acid compositions of milk phosphatidylcholine, phosphatidylethanolamine and sphingomyelin are shown in Table 25. Accompanying these are analyses by Boatman et al.[33] on phosphatidylethanolamine and phosphatidylserine and by Bracco et al.[39] on phosphatidylinositol. The differences in composition between the samples of phosphatidylethanolamine and -serine can be attributed to nutritional, environmental and genetic effects.

Hay and Morrison[133] have thoroughly analyzed both the fatty acid composition and the structure of milk phosphatidylethanolamine and -choline. The data, presented in Table 26, reveal that the structure usually observed in these phospholipids from other sources, saturates in the 1-position and unsaturates, medium chain length and branched acids in the 2-position, did not occur to the same extent with the milk compounds. This "scrambling" might have been caused by mixing of exogenous and endogenous acids during synthesis. Phytanic acid was found only in the 1-position of the two phospholipids. The steric hindrance presented by the four methyl branches apparently prevents acylation at the 2-position. The fairly even distribution of monoenoic acids between the two positions (Table 26) is altered when the *trans* isomers are considered (Table 27), as a marked asymmetry appears with 18:1 between the 1- and 2-positions of phosphatidylethanolamine, but not the phosphatidylcholine. The *trans* isomers are apparently handled biologically the same as the equivalent saturates because the latter have almost the same distribution (see Table 26). There were no appreciable differences in distribution of *cis* or *trans* positional isomers between positions 1 and 2 in either phospholipids (Table 28). Another structural asymmetry is seen in Table 29 where *cis,cis* nonconjugated 18:2s were located mostly

TABLE 25. *Fatty Acid Composition (Mole%) of Various Bovine Milk Phospholipids*[a]

Fatty acid	Phosphatidyl ethanolamine		Phosphatidyl choline	Sphingomyelin	Phosphatidyl serine		Phosphatidyl inositol
12:0	tr	—[b]	0.7	0.3	3.6	1.6[b]	—[c]
14:0	1.5	1.0	8.4	2.5	12.5	5.2	4.7
15:0	0.5	—	2.1	0.4	—	—	1.3
16:0	11.7	11.0	36.4	22.1	31.7	15.0	29.8
16:1	2.1	1.1	0.6	0.8	—	—	—
17:0	0.9	—	0.9	0.6	—	—	—
18:0	10.5	13.0	11.1	4.5	13.0	30.0	31.8
18:1	46.7	61.0	25.7	5.0	32.9	38.0	10.8
18:2	12.4	12.0	5.3	0.9	4.9	7.3	6.9
18:3	3.4	2.1	1.1	—	—	3.2	2.5
20:3	1.4	—	1.0	—	—	—	—
20:4	1.9	—	0.7	—	—	—	—
22:0	—	—	—	14.7	—	—	3.9
23:0	—	—	—	27.0	—	—	—
24:0	—	—	—	14.8	—	—	—

[a] Adapted from ref. 245. Minor acids omitted.
[b] Adapted from ref. 33. Minor acids omitted.
[c] From ref. 39, 3.8% 20:0 omitted.

in the 2-position in both phospholipids. It appears that one or more *trans* double bonds in the 18:2s hinders the acylation of these acids to the 2-position.

Hay and Morrison[133] did not neglect the alkyl and alkenyl ethers in milk phospholipids, finding 4% of the latter in phosphatidylethanolamine and 1.3% in phosphatidylcholine. The alkyl and alkenyl composition of phosphatidylcholine is given in Table 30. *Trans* isomers were not found. The authors postulated that the branched chain compounds in the alkenyl ethers were derived from rumen microbial lipids.

TABLE 26. *Composition of the Fatty Acids (mole %) in the 1- and 2-Positions of Bovine Milk Phosphatidylethanolamine and Phosphatidylcholine*[a]

	Fatty acid	Phosphatidylethanolamine 1-position	2-position	Total	Phosphatidylcholine 1-position	2-position	Total
	10:0				0.2	0.3	0.25
	11:0				0.1	tr	0.05
	12:0	tr	0.8	0.2	0.3	1.2	0.75
	12:1	tr	tr	tr		0.4	0.2
	13:0	tr	0.3	0.15	tr	0.1	0.05
iso	14:0		0.1	0.05	0.5	0.1	0.3
	14:0	1.3	1.2	1.25	4.1	12.4	8.25
	14:1	0.1	0.1	0.1	0.1	0.1	0.1
iso	15:0	0.1	0.1	0.1	0.2	0.7	0.45
anteiso	15:0	0.1	0.2	0.15	0.2	0.7	0.45
	15:0	0.2	0.5	0.35	1.5	1.9	1.7
	15:1	0.1	0.1	0.1	0.1	0.3	0.2
iso	16:0	0.1	0.1	0.1	0.4	0.6	0.5
	16:0	10.7	4.6	7.65	34.4	27.7	31.05
	16:1	0.8	1.2	1.0	1.2	0.7	0.95
iso	17:0	0.1	0.2	0.15	0.6	0.7	0.65
anteiso	17:0	0.2	0.3	0.25	0.7	0.7	0.7
	17:0	0.8	0.5	0.65	1.3	0.4	0.85
	17:1	0.2	1.1	0.65	0.5	1.0	0.75
	18:0	27.7	1.3	14.5	21.5	3.2	12.35
	18:1	52.0	61.2	56.6	25.5	36.7	31.1
	18:2	1.7	13.9	7.8	2.3	4.8	3.55
conj.	18:2 (c,t)[b]	1.1	0.7	0.9	0.6	0.7	0.65
conj.	18:2 (t,t)	0.7	0.7	0.7	0.4	0.3	0.35
	18:3	0.8	4.2	2.5	0.8	1.0	0.9
	19:0	0.2		0.1	0.8	0.5	0.65
	19:1		1.0	0.05	0.1	0.1	0.1
	20:0 br 4	0.1		0.05	1.0		0.5
	20:0	0.3	0.2	0.25	0.3	0.3	0.3
	20:1	0.1	0.4	0.25	0.1	0.3	0.2
	20:3		1.0	0.5		0.3	0.15
	20:4		1.4	0.7		0.4	0.2
	21:0	0.1		0.05	tr		tr
Unknowns		0.4	3.5	1.05	0.2	1.4	0.8

[a]From Hay and Morrison.[133]
[b]Abbreviations: conj. 18:2 (c,t) = *cis, trans* conjugated octadecadienoate, conj. 18:2 (t,t) = *trans, trans* conjugated octadecadienoate, 20:0 br 4 = phytanate, tr = trace amounts present.

TABLE 27. *Trans Isomers (wt %) in the Monoenoic Fatty Acids in the 1- and 2-Positions of Bovine Milk Phosphatidylethanolamine and Phosphatidylcholine*[a]

Fatty acid	Phosphatidylethanolamine		Phosphatidylcholine	
	1-position	2-position	1-position	2-position
16:1	11.3	9.3	24.2, 26.0	20.1, 25.4
17:1	1.9	tr	2.1	tr, tr
18:1	15.0	0.9	25.7, 26.2	1.3, 1.1

[a]Hay and Morrison.[133]

Bracco et al.[39] have determined the fatty acid composition of milk fat globule membranes phospholipids and these are tabulated in Table 31. There were some major differences between the fatty acid contents of these phospholipids as compared to the phospholipids of milk in general (Table 25). For example, the membrane phos-

TABLE 28. *Distribution of Double Bonds (wt %) in CIS and TRANS Monoenoic Fatty Acids in the 1- and 2-Positions of Bovine Milk Phosphatidylethanolamine and Phosphatidylcholine Compared with Triglyceride*[a]

Position of double bond from carboxyl	16:1			17:1			18:1				
	1-PC	2-PC	TG	1-PC	2-PC	TG	1-PE	2-PE	1-PC	2-PC	TG
cis isomers											
5			<1								
6	2	4	1		4	2			1		
7	8	6	7	3	2	2			<1	1	<1
8	1	1	<1	17	14	22	<1	<1	1	1	1
9	82	85	87	80	79	70	95	95	95	98	96
10	2	<1	1		tr	2		<1	<1		<1
11	4	2	3		1	2	3	5	3	1	3
12	1	1	1				<1		1		
13	<1		<1								
trans isomers											
5	<1		1								
6	4	1	5								
7	1	1	3					1		<1	1
8	1	tr	3				<1	tr	<1	<1	2
9	63	69	46				17	21	5	5	4
10	<1	2	4				3	8	1	1	4
11	4	6	8				53	48	57	46	45
12	10	5	12				4	4	3	4	5
13	9	10	9				7	7	8	12	9
14	6	6	9				7	2	9	9	9
15							5	4	8	8	8
16							4	5	7	7	13

[a]Hay and Morrison.[133]

TABLE 29. *Composition of Octadecadienoic Fatty Acids (wt %) in the 1- and 2- Positions of Bovine Milk Phosphatidylethanolamine and Phosphatidylcholine*[a]

Octadecadienoate	Phosphatidylethanolamine		Phosphatidylcholine	
	1-position	2-position	1-position	2-position
cis, trans conjugated	1.1	0.7	0.6	0.7
trans, trans conjugated	0.7	0.7	0.4	0.3
cis, trans and trans, trans nonconjugated	0.3	1.8	0.5	0.6
cis, cis nonconjugated	1.4	12.1	2.0	4.2

[a]Hay and Morrison.[133]

TABLE 30. *Composition (wt %) of the Alkyl and Alkenyl Ethers in Bovine Milk Phosphatidyl choline*[a]

Aliphatic chain		Alkyl ethers	Alkenyl ethers	Aliphatic chain		Alkyl ethers	Alkenyl ethers
br	13:0	—	0.2		16:1	0.7	4.6
	13:0	1.0	0.2	iso	17:0	1.2	1.6
br	14:0A	0.8	8.2	anteiso	17:0	1.5	3.8
br	14:0B	1.2	—		17:0	1.5	2.4
	14:0	3.6	3.4		17:1	0.6	—
iso	15:0	1.4	6.7	iso	18:0	0.9	0.4
anteiso	15:0	2.4	20.1		18:0	25.5	4.8
	15:0	2.8	5.4		18:1	10.8	0.8
	15:1	0.3	—	iso	19:0	2.4	1.3
iso	16:0	1.0	3.2	anteiso	19:0	±	2.5
	16:0	30.4	30.4		19:0	0.8	—

[a]Adapted from ref. 133.

TABLE 31. *Fatty Acid Composition of Phospholipids from the Bovine Milk Fat Globule Membrane*[a]

Fatty acids	PE[b]	PC	Sph	LPC	PI	PS
			wt. %			
12:0	1.1	1.4	3.2	1.5	—	—
14:0	7.6	8.0	7.1	3.9	4.7	17.1
15:0	—	—	1.7	8.6	1.3	—
16:0	31.6	12.8	17.8	13.6	29.8	15.6
18:0	15.1	11.1	14.6	21.7	31.8	29.7
18:1	17.3	31.2	30.7	28.6	10.8	14.6
18:2	6.5	3.2	4.7	5.1	6.9	3.1
18:3	5.5	4.3	2.8	—	2.5	—
20:0	1.1	—	5.1	—	4.5	3.8
20:4	1.2	1.5	—	—	—	—
22:0	1.8	—	4.6	4.7	—	3.9

[a]Adapted from ref. 39.
[b]PE—phosphatidylethanolamine, etc.

phatidylethenolamine contained more saturated acids than the phosphatidylethanolamine from total milk lipid. However, such comparisons are made with greatest validity using the same sample of milk.

5. Sphingolipids

Morrison[245] presented earlier data on the fatty acid composition of these lipids. In a later paper Morrison and Hay[248] described the isolation and analyses of milk sphingomyelin, glucosylceramide and lactosylceramide. The long-chain bases were similar in all compounds consisting of normal, iso and anteiso saturated and unsaturated dihydroxy bases (Table 32). The bases present in largest quantity were 18:1, 16:1, 17:1, 16:0, 18:0, iso 18:1 and iso 17:1, with many branched chain bases occurring in smaller amounts. The major fatty acids both normal and 2-hydroxy were usually 22:0, 23:0 and 24:0 with some variations (Table 33). Hydroxy acids were observed to comprise less than 1% of the total acids. The *trans* acid content of total sphingolipids were 43–51%, higher than in the corresponding milk fat with the 18:1, 22:1, 23:1, 24:1 and 25:1 isomers present in sphingomyelin, glucosyl ceramide and lactosyl ceramide. In sphingomyelin there was a trend with high *trans* contents in 18:1 (94.2%) to lower amounts in 25:1 (7.1%). Morrison and Hay[248] analyzed the *cis* and *trans* 23:1, 24:1 and 25:1 acids of sphingomyelin for positional isomers. The results (Table 34) show that the *cis* acids were similar to the *cis* 18:1s in milk fat (Table 18), but not the *trans* acids, with decreased amounts of Δ-9 isomers and much larger quantities of Δ-11. The latter is unusual, but might be explained by the positional isomerization known to accompany elaidinization during hydrogenation.

TABLE 32. *Composition (wt %) of Dihydroxy Long-chain Bases in Bovine Milk Sphingolipids*[a]

Base	Sphingo-myelin	Glucosyl ceramide	Lactosyl ceramide	Base	Sphingo-myelin	Glucosyl ceramide	Lactosyl ceramide
12:0	0.1	—	0.2	12:1	0.5	0.3	0.3
14:0	0.1	0.5	0.4	13:1	0.4	0.5	0.7
15:0	0.1	0.8	0.6	iso 14:1	0.2	0.3	0.2
iso 16:0	—	0.3	0.5	14:1	1.3	1.6	1.5
16:0	8.2	2.1	3.6	iso 15:1	0.2	0.3	0.6
iso 17:0	0.2	—	0.6	anteiso 15:1	0.4	0.6	0.3
anteiso 17:0	0.2	0.5	0.9	15:1	0.5	1.5	1.2
17:0	1.1	1.0	1.6	iso 16:1	—	0.2	0.2
iso 18:0	0.4	0.8	0.3	16 1	21.0	10.4	11.6
18 0	5.9	2.0	4.9	iso 17 1	1.2	0.8	1.3
iso 19 0	0.3	—	—	anteiso 17 1	0.8	1.1	1.4
anteiso 19 0	0.2	—	—	17 1	6.4	4.7	3.9
19 0	0.2	1.3	1.5	iso 18 1	8.9	6.7	7.7
iso 20 0	0.2	1.6	1.4	18 1	33.5	48.1	37.6
20 0	0.6	2.7	6.2	iso 19 1	1.8	2.2	2.0
				anteiso 19 1	3.5	3.2	2.4
				19 1	0.8	2.0	2.2
				20 1	0.8	1.9	1.5

[a]Adapted from ref. 248.

TABLE 33. *Fatty Acids (wt %) of Bovine Milk Sphingolipids*[a]

Fatty acid	Sphingomyelin Normal	Sphingomyelin Hydroxy	Glucosylceramide Normal	Glucosylceramide Hydroxy	Lactosylceramide Normal	Lactosylceramide Hydroxy
12:0	0.1	—	—	—	0.1	—
14:0	0.4	1.6	1.0	2.8	0.3	0.6
15:0	0.1	—	0.3	—	0.1	—
16:0	7.8	9.2	9.3	12.6	7.7	10.5
16:1	—	0.8	1.4	—	0.3	—
17:0	0.3	1.1	1.3	1.3	0.2	1.1
18:0	1.6	6.2	13.7	8.4	3.3	3.7
18:1	0.2	0.7	12.2	—	1.3	—
18:2	0.2	—	2.0	—	0.2	—
19:0	0.2	0.6	1.3	—	0.2	—
20:0	0.6	0.6	0.9	4.5	1.1	1.2
21:0	0.9	2.0	1.2	1.3	1.4	0.9
21:1	—	—	0.1	—	—	—
22:0	20.7	17.2	17.0	16.7	24.9	15.4
22:1	0.7	—	0.9	—	0.6	—
23:0	30.4	31.5	22.0	31.0	29.5	26.9
23:1	5.0	2.5	3.4	1.7	6.6	6.3
24:0	22.8	21.8	9.9	19.7	16.5	29.5
24:1	4.0	1.5	2.1	—	3.7	4.1
25:0	1.6	1.9	—	—	0.7	—
25:1	1.6	1.0	—	—	1.4	—
26:0	0.8	—	—	—	—	—

[a]Adapted from ref. 248.

In an earlier paper, Morrison[244] reported that he found no saturated trihydroxy bases (t:o) in bovine milk sphingolipids. However, after a more thorough search a t:o enriched fraction was isolated from milk sphingomyelin (1% of the total).[246] This fraction contained the trihydroxy bases listed in Table 35. The composition of the

TABLE 34. *Positional Isomers (wt %) of* CIS *and* TRANS *Monoenoic Acids from Bovine Milk Sphingolipids*[a]

Position of double bond	cis isomers 23:1	cis isomers 24:1	cis isomers 25:1	trans isomers 23:1	trans isomers 24:1	trans isomers 25:1
6		0.3			0.6	
7	1.2	0.1	0.7	1.2	0.8	1.2
8	2.3	1.0	3.0	2.1	7.5	2.3
9	79.0	96.5	92.5	59.6	21.1	3.6
10	5.2	1.0	2.8	9.3	6.5	3.6
11	8.6		1.0	1.7	24.4	45.3
12	2.3	0.3		8.9	5.7	4.7
13	0.7			2.5	11.3	8.8
14	0.7			12.4	19.6	8.8
15				3.2	3.2	8.4
16						13.0

[a]Reference 248.

t:o bases are similar to the d:1 or total hydrogenated bases. Therefore, Morrison suggested that the cow is able to synthesize t:o bases from the same fatty acids used for synthesis of dihydroxy bases. Later Morrison[247] concluded after analyzing the long-chain bases in the sphingolipids of bovine milk and kidney, rumen bacteria, rumen protozoa, hay and concentrate that the milk and kidney sphingomyelin bases were not of dietary origin. He further decided that bovine tissues synthesize straight and branched saturated dihydroxy, (d:o), d:1⁴ᵗ and t:o long-chain bases.

TABLE 35. *Composition of Long-chain Bases in Bovine Milk Sphingomyelin*[a]

	Chain length	d:0	d:1	t:0	Total hydrog.
	14	0.9 ± 0.2	0.5 ± 0.0		
	16	54.0 ± 1.5	26.4 ± 1.6	22.0 ± 1.5	27.4 ± 0.6
iso	17	0.9 ± 0.0	1.4 ± 0.1	2.0 ± 0.3	1.3 ± 0.1
	17	6.6 ± 0.2	8.5 ± 0.3	10.7 ± 0.5	8.9 ± 0.2
iso	18	4.3 ± 0.2	11.7 ± 0.3	9.2 ± 0.3	11.2 ± 0.1
	18	29.6 ± 1.3	45.8 ± 0.7	49.0 ± 1.2	45.5 ± 0.5
iso	19	0.8 ± 0.1	1.1 ± 0.2	1.9 ± 0.5	1.3 ± 0.1
anteiso	19	1.3 ± 0.2	3.3 ± 0.4	3.8 ± 0.6	2.9 ± 0.2
	19	0.5 ± 0.0	1.0 ± 0.1	1.4 ± 0.4	1.1 ± 0.1
	20	1.1 ± 0.1	0.3 ± 0.0		0.4 ± 0.0
Percentage of total bases		17	82	<1	100

[a]Values are given as uncorrected weight percentages ±1 standard deviation. Sizes of samples were d:0 = 6, d:1 = 9, t:0 = 10. Reference 244.

Kayser and Patton[166] also identified the components of milk glucosyl and lactosyl ceramides (cerebrosides). Fatty acids of the cerebrosides bound to the fat globule membrane were mainly 20:0–25:0, 74.0 and 58.0% long-chain for glucosyl and lactosyl ceramides, respectively. In skim milk, the proportions were lower with 28.0% and 17.0% sat of long-chain acids in the two ceramides. Fujino and Fujishima[110] found 16 fatty acids in the free ceramides of bovine milk, with 90% consisting of 16:0, 22:0, 23:0 and 24:0. Seven accompanying sphingosine bases were observed with the C-16, 16-methyl-C-17 and C-18 compounds accounting for 83% of the total. According to the authors this was the first isolation of ceramide, in free form, from bovine milk.

The partitioning of fatty acids observed by Kayser and Patton has important implications with regard to the milk component from which polar lipids are extracted. Patton and Keenan[275] had found that 42 and 58% of the lipid phosphorus in milk occurred in skim milk lipoprotein and in the milk fat globule membrane, respectively. The two sources of lipid phosphorus contained the same phospholipids, which in most cases had similar fatty acid compositions. Nevertheless, the varying compositions of cerebrosides from the two sources, both from the same milk, indicate that the two sources are different in composition and are not, therefore, representative samples of milk polar lipids as in fresh whole milk.

Huang[145] analyzed the fatty acids of milk gangliosides, finding the following amounts (%): 14:0, 4.2; 16:0, 20.2; 16:1, 2.8; 18:0, 18.1; 18:1, 36.6; 18:2, 7.8; 20:0, 3.0 and 20:4, 6.1. Hydroxy acids were not detected. The sphingosine base contents (%) were: sphinganines; C-16, 10; C-18, 5 and sphingenines; C-16, 20 and C-18, 32. Several branched bases were also noted but not further identified. The composition of the gangliosides is quite different from that of milk sphingomyelin and other glycolipids, suggesting perhaps, selectivity during biosynthesis.

6. Sterol esters

Keenan and Patton[178] isolated and identified the cholesterol esters from cow, sow and goat milk and mammary tissue. The fatty acid compositions of the esters from the cow are tabulated in Table 36. The authors commented that the concentrations of monounsaturated, other than 18:1, and odd-numbered fatty acids in the cholesterol esters were greater than those found in milk triacylglycerols. For example, only traces of 13:1 are found in the latter.

TABLE 36. *Fatty Acid Composition of Cholesterol Esters from Bovine Milk*[a]

Fatty acid	Wt%	Fatty acid	Wt%
10:0	2.9	15:1	2.6
10:1	0.3	16:0	26.9
12:0	4.1	16:1	11.9
12:1	0.2	17:0	tr
13:0	tr	17:1	ND
13:1	11.0	18:0	6.7
14:0	6.9	18:1	13.7
14:1	0.5	18:2	10.1
15:0	2.1		

[a]Adapted from ref. 178.

C. Summary

The major lipid classes and components of milk have apparently been identified and future research will probably involve the minor lipids, so-called because the quantities are small. Undoubtedly many additional fatty acids are present, dependent perhaps on what types of plants the cow consumes and on variations in the rumen fermentation. Some may be ephemeral. Thus many intriguing problems of isolation and identification remain.

The complexity of milk lipids is best observed in Table 37, where we have summarized the fatty acid composition of milk lipids and arrived at a total of 437! If we include 33 sphingosine and sphingenine dihydroxy long-chain bases, 8 trihydroxy bases, 70 alkyl ethers and 50 alkenyl ethers, the total of all is a staggering 598. An estimate of all the individual lipid molecular species would give a number in the very high thousands if all TGs were included. Bovine milk, therefore, contains the most complex known lipid.

TABLE 37. *Fatty Acid Composition of Milk Lipids as of January 1974*[a]

Number	Type	Identity
	Saturates	
27	normal	2–28;
71	monobranched	11–28; 11–19 three or more positional isomers
18	multibranched	16–28
	Monoenes	
57	*cis*	10–26, except for 11:1, positional isomers of 12:1, 14:1, 16:1–18:1 and 23:1–15:1
58	*trans*	12–14, 16–24; positional isomers of 14:1, 16:1–18:1 and 23:1–25:1
42	Dienes	14–26 evens only; *cis, cis, cis, trans* or *trans, cis* and *trans, trans*, geometric isomers, unconjugated and conjugated and positional isomers
	Polyenes	
10	tri-	18, 20, 22; geometric positional, conjugated and unconjugated isomers
5	tetra-	18, 20, 22; positional isomers
2	penta-	20, 22
1	hexa-	22
	Keto (oxo)	
38	saturate	10, 12, 14, 15–20, 22, 24; positional isomers
21	unsaturate	14, 16, 18; positional isomers of carbonyl and double bond
	Hydroxy	
16	2-position	14:0, 16:0–26:0; 16:1, 18:1, 21:1, 23:1, 24:1, 25:1
9	4 & 5 position	10:0–16:0, 12:Δ-6 and 12:1-Δ-9
60	other positions	
	Cyclic	
2	hexyl,	9 and 11; terminal cyclohexyl
437		

[a]Compiled from refs. 2, 89, 127, 151, 157, 159, 245, 248, 314, 322, 350, 362 and 370.

ACKNOWLEDGEMENTS

Portions of the research discussed herein were supported by grants of the National Institutes of Health (HL 03632) and programs of the Pennsylvania and Storrs Agricultural Experiment Stations. We thank R. D. McCarthy and P. S. Dimick for reviewing the manuscript, Bridget Stemberger for preparation of photomicrographs and Lori Bathgate for typing the manuscripts. S. Patton is grateful to E. G. Trams, A. A. Benson and T. W. Keenan for stimulating discussions on the subject of membranes.

REFERENCES

1. ACKMAN, R. G., *Progress in the Chemistry of Fats and Other Lipids*, Vol. 12, p. 165. R. T. Holman, ed. Oxford: Pergamon Press (1972).
2. ACKMAN, R. G. and HANSEN, R. P., *Lipids*, **2**, 357–362 (1967).
3. ACKMAN, R. G., HOOPER, S. N. and HANSEN, R. P., *Lipids*, **7**, 683–691 (1972).
4. AHRENS, R. A., and LUICK, J. R., *J. Dairy Sci.*, **47**, 849–854 (1964).
5. ALEXANDER, K. M. and LUSENA, C. V., *J. Dairy Sci.*, **44**, 1414–1419 (1961).
6. AMBRON, R. T. and PIERINGER, R. A., *Form and Function of Phospholipids*, p. 289. G. B. Ansell, R. M. C. Dawson and J. N. Hawthorne, eds. Amsterdam: Elsevier (1973).
7. ANNISON, E. F. and LINZELL, J. L. *J. Physiol.*, **175**, 372–385 (1964).

8. Annison, E. F., Linzell, J. L., Fazakerely, S. and Nichols, B. W., *Biochem. J.*, **102**, 637–647 (1967).
9. Ansell, G. B., Dawson, R. M. C. and Hawthorne, J. N., eds., *Form and Function of Phospholipids*. Amsterdam: Elsevier (1973).
10. Assn. Off. Agr. Chemists, *Official Methods of Analysis*, 10th ed., p. 224 (1965).
11. Baldwin, R. L., *J. Dairy Sci.*, **52**, 729–736 (1969).
12. Ballard, F. J., Hanson, R. W. and Kronfield, D. S., *Fed. Proc.*, **28**, 218–231 (1969).
13. Bangham, A. D., *Ann. Rev. Biochem.*, **41**, 753–775 (1972).
14. Bangham, A. D. and Horne, R. W., *J. Mol. Biol.*, **8**, 660–668 (1964).
15. Bargmann, W., Fleischauer, K. and Knoop, A., *Z. Zellforsch.*, **53**, 545–568 (1961).
16. Bargmann, W. and Knoop, A., *Z. Zellforsch.*, **49**, 344–388 (1959).
17. Barry, J. M., Bartley, W., Linzell, J. L. and Robinson, D. S., *Biochem. J.*, **89**, 6–11 (1963).
18. Bauer, H., *J. Dairy Sci.*, **55**, 1375–1387 (1972).
19. Bauman, D. E. and Davis, C. L., *Lactation: A Comprehensive Treatise*, Vol. II. B. L. Larson and V. R. Smith, eds. New York and London: Academic Press (1974).
20. Bauman, D. E., Engle, D. L., Mellenberger, R. W. and Davis, C. L., *J. Dairy Sci.*, **56**, 1520–1525 (1973).
21. Baumrucker, C. R. and Keenan, T. W., *J. Dairy Sci.*, **56**, 1092–1094 (1973).
22. Baumrucker, C. R. and Keenan, T. W., *J. Dairy Sci.*, **57**, 24–31 (1974).
23. Beery, K. E., Hood, L. F. and Patton, S., *J. Dairy Sci.*, **54**, 911–912 (1971).
24. Bergelson, L. D., *Progress in the Chemistry of Fats and Other Lipids*, Vol. 10 (3), p. 239. R. T. Holman, ed. Oxford: Pergamon Press (1969).
25. Berlin, E., Lakshamanan, S., Kliman, P. G. and Pallansch, M. J., *Biochemistry*, **6**, 1388–1394 (1967).
26. Bickerstaffe, R. and Johnson, A. R., *Brit. J. Nutr.*, **27**, 561–570 (1972).
27. Bickerstaffe, R., Linzell, J. L., Morris, L. J. and Annison, E. F., *Biochem. J.*, **117**, 36 p. (1970).
28. Bilheimer, D. W., Eisenberg, S. and Levy, R. I., *Biochim. Biophys. Acta*, **260**, 212–221 (1972).
29. Bingham, E. W., Farrell, H. M. and Basch, I. J., *J. Biol. Chem.*, **247**, 8193–8194 (1972).
30. Birkinshaw, M. and Falconer, I. R., *J. Endocr.*, **55**, 323–334 (1972).
31. Bishop, C., Davies, T., Glascock, R. F., and Welch V. A., *Biochem. J.*, **113**, 629–632 (1969).
32. Bitman, J. L., Dryden, L. P., Goering, H. K., Wrenn, T. R., Yoncoskie, R. A. and Edmonson, L. F., *J. Amer. Oil Chemists' Soc.*, **50**, 93–98 (1973).
33. Boatman, V. E., Patton, S. and Parsons, J. G., *J. Dairy Sci.*, **52**, 256–258 (1969).
34. Body, R. J., *FEBS Letters*, **27**, 5–8 (1972).
35. Boguslawski, W. and Wrobel, J., *Nature*, **247**, 210–211 (1974).
36. Bolis, L. and Keynes, R. D., eds., *Role of Membranes in Secretory Processes*. New York: Elsevier (1972).
37. Boot, L. M., *Int. J. Cancer*, **5**, 167–175 (1970).
38. Boudreau, A. and deMan, J. M., *Biochim. Biophys. Acta*, **98**, 47–52 (1965).
39. Bracco, U., Hidalgo, J. and Bohren, H., *J. Dairy Sci.*, **55**, 165–172 (1972).
40. Bragdon, J. H., Havel, R. J. and Boyle, E., *J. Lab. Clin. Med.*, **48**, 36–42 (1956).
41. Breach, R. A., Dils, R. and Watts, R., *J. Dairy Res.*, **40**, 273–287 (1973).
42. Breckenridge, W. C., and Kuksis A., *J. Lipid Res.*, **9**, 388–393 (1968).
43. Breckenridge, W. C. and Kuksis, A., *Lipids*, **4**, 197–204 (1969).
44. Bretscher, M. S., *Science*, **181**, 622–629 (1973).
45. Brew. K., Vanaman, T. C. and Hill, R. L., *Proc. Nat. Acad. Sci.*, **59**, 491–497 (1968).
46. Brewington, C. R., Caress, E. A. and Schwartz, D. P., *J. Lipid Res.*, **11**, 355–361 (1970).
47. Brian, B. L., Gracy, R. W. and Scholes, V. E., *J. Chromat.*, **66**, 138–140 (1972).
48. Brink, M. F. and Kritchevsky, D., eds., *Dairy Lipids and Lipid Metabolism*. Westport, Connecticut: Avi Publishing Co. (1968).
49. Brockerhoff, H., *J. Lipid Res.*, **6**, 10–15 (1965).
50. Brockerhoff, H., *Lipids*, **6**, 942–956 (1971).
51. Brockerhoff, H. and Jensen, R. G., *Lipolytic Enzymes*. New York and London: Academic Press (1974).
52. Brodbeck, U. and Ebner, K. E., *J. Biol. Chem.*, **241**, 762–764 (1966).
53. Brunner, J. R., *Fundamentals of Dairy Chemistry*, p. 403. B. H. Webb and A. H. Johnson, eds. Westport, Connecticut: Avi Publishing Co. (1965).
54. Brunner, J. R., *Structural and Functional Aspects of Lipoproteins in Living Systems*, p. 545. E. Tria and A. M. Scanu, eds. New York and London: Academic Press (1969).
55. Buckheim, W. and Welsch, U., *Neth. Milk Dairy J.*, **27**, 163–180 (1973).
56. Buehring, G. C., *J. Natl. Cancer Inst.*, **49**, 1433–1434 (1972).
57. Butler, J. E., Winter, A. J. and Wagner, G. C., *J. Dairy Sci.*, **54**, 1309–1340 (1971).

REFERENCES

58. CALL, F. L. II and RUBERT, M. J., *Lipid Res.*, **14**, 466–474 (1973).
59. CAREY, E. M. and DILS, R., *Biochem. J.*, **126**, 1005–1007 (1972).
60. CAREY, E. M., DILS, R. and HANSEN, H. J. M., *Biochem. J.*, **117**, 633–635 (1970).
61. CHAN, P. -C. and COHEN, L. A., *J. Natl. Cancer Inst.* **52**, 25–30 (1974).
62. CHEN, M. -H. and LARSON, B. L., *J. Dairy Sci.*, **54**, 842–846 (1971).
63. CHESTERTON, C. J., *J. Biol. Chem.*, **243**, 1147–1151 (1968).
64. CHEVALIER, F. and LUTTON, C., *Nature New Biology*, **242**, 61–62 (1973).
65. CHRISTIE, W. W., *Topics in Lipid Chemistry*, Vol. 1, p. 1. F. D. Gunstone, ed. London: Logos Press, Paul Elek, Ltd. (1970).
66. CHRISTOPHERSON, S. W. and GLASS, R. L., *J. Dairy Sci.*, **52**, 1289–1290 (1969).
67. CLARENBURG, R. and CHAIKOFF, I. L., *J. Lipid Res.*, **7**, 27–37 (1966).
68. COCCODRILLI, G. D. Ph.D. Thesis, The Pennsylvania State University (1971).
69. CONNOR, W. E. and LIN, D. S., *Amer. J. Physiol.*, **213**, 1353–1358 (1967).
70. DAVIS, C. L. and BAUMAN, D. E., *Lactation: A Comprehensive Treatise*, Vol. II. B. L. Larson and V. R. Smith, eds. New York and London: Academic Press (1974).
71. DAVIS, C. L. and BROWN, R. E., *Physiology of Digestion and Metabolism in the Ruminant*, A. T. Phillipson, ed. Newcastle upon Tyne: Oriel Press (1970).
72. DAWSON, R. M. C. and RHODES, D. N., eds. *Metabolism and Physiological Significance of Lipids*. New York, London, Sydney: John Wiley (1964).
73. DAY, A. J., WAHLQUIST, M. L. and CAMPBELL, D. J., *Atherosclerosis*, **11**, 301–320 (1970).
74. DEIS, R. P., *Nature*, **229**, 568 (1971).
75. DELOUIS, C. and DENAMUR, R., *J. Endocr.*, **52**, 311–319 (1972).
76. DEMAN, J. M., *Zeitschrift fur Ernahrungswissenschaft*, **5**, 1–4 (1964).
77. DENAMUR, R., *Ann. Endocr., Paris*, **22**, 768–776 (1961).
78. DENNIS, E. A. and KENNEDY, E. P., *J. Lipid Res.*, **13**, 263–267 (1972).
79. DICKES, G. J. and NICHOLAS, P. V., *J. Assoc. Publ. Analysts*, **10**, 87–98 (1972).
80. DILS, R. and CLARK, B., *Biochem. J.*, **84**, 19 p. (1962).
81. DIMICK, P. S., MCCARTHY, R. D. and PATTON, S., *Biochim. Biophys. Acta*, **116**, 159–162 (1966).
82. DIMICK, P. S., MCCARTHY, R. D. and PATTON, S., *Physiology of Digestion and Metabolism in the Ruminant*, pp. 529–541. A. T. Phillipson, ed. Newcastle upon Tyne: Oriel Press (1970).
83. DIMICK, P. S. and PATTON, S., *J. Dairy Sci.*, **48**, 444–449 (1965).
84. DIMICK, P. S., WALKER, N. J. and PATTON, S., *Biochem. J.*, **111**, 395–399 (1969).
85. DIMICK, P. S., WALKER, N. J. and PATTON, S., *J. Agr. Food Chem.*, **17**, 649–655 (1969).
86. DOWBEN, R. M., BRUNNER, J. R. and PHILPOTT, D. E., *Biochim. Biophys. Acta*, **135**, 1–10 (1967).
87. EASTER, D. J., *Lipids*, **6**, 645–648 (1971).
88. EASTER, D. J., PATTON, S. and MCCARTHY, R. D., *Lipids*, **6**, 844–849 (1971).
89. EGGE, H., MURAWSKI, U., RYHAGE, R., GYORGY, P., CHATRANON, W. and ZILLIKIN, F. *Chem. Phys. Lipids*, **8**, 42–55 (1972).
90. EISENBERG, S., BILHEIMER, D. W., LEVY, R. I. and LINDGREN, F. T. *Biochim. Biophys. Acta*, **326**, 361–377 (1973).
91. EISENBERG, S. and RACHMILEWITZ, D., *Biochim. Biophys. Acta*, **326**, 378–405 (1973).
92. EISENBERG, S., STEIN, Y. and STEIN, O., *Biochim. Biophys. Acta*, **176**, 557–569 (1969).
93. ELLINGBOE, J. and STEINBERG, D., *Biochim. Biophys. Acta*, **270**, 92–102 (1972).
94. EMERY, R. S., *J. Dairy Sci.*, **56**, 1187–1195 (1973).
95. EVANS, L. and PATTON, S., *J. Dairy Sci.*, **45**, 589–594 (1962).
96. EVANS, L., PATTON, S. and MCCARTHY, R. D., *J. Dairy Sci.* **44**, 475–482 (1961).
97. EVANS, W. H. and GURD, J. W., *Biochem. J.*, **133**, 189–199 (1973).
98. FALCONER, I. R., ed. *Lactation*. University Park and London: The Pennsylvania State University Press (1971).
99. FARRELL, H. M., Jr., *J. Dairy Sci.*, **56**, 1195–1206 (1973).
100. FELL, H. B., *J. Embryol. exp. Morph.*, **10**, 389–409 (1962).
101. FLANAGAN, V. P. and FERRETTI, A., *J. Lipid Res.*, **14**, 306–311 (1973).
102. FORSS, D. A., *Progress in the Chemistry of Fats and Other Lipids*, Vol. 13 (4), pp. 177–258. R. T. Holman, ed. Oxford: Pergamon Press (1972).
103. FORSYTH, I. A., *J. Dairy Res.*, **38**, 419–445 (1971).
104. FORTE, G. M., NICHOLS, A. V. and GLAESER, R. M., *Chem. Phys. Lipids*, **2**, 396–408 (1968).
105. FORTE, T. M., NICHOLS, A. V., GONG, E. L., LUX, S. and LEVI, R. I., *Biochim. Biophys. Acta*, **248**, 381–386 (1971).
106. FOX, C. F., ed., *Membrane Research*. New York and London: Academic Press (1972).
107. FREDERICKSON, D. S. and GORDON, R. S., Jr., *Physiol. Rev.*, **38**, 585–630 (1958).
108. FREDERICKSON, D. S., LEVY, R. I., JONES, E., BONNELL, M. and ERNST, M., *Dietary Management of Hyperlipoproteinemia*, p. 14. Bethesda, Maryland: National Heart and Lung Institute (1971).
109. FREDERICKSON, D. S., LEVY, R. I. and LEES, R., *New Engl. J. Med.*, **276**, 34–44, 94–103, 148–156, 215–281 (1967).

110. Fujino, Y. and Fujishima, T., *J. Dairy Res.*, **39**, 11–14 (1972)
111. Galli, C., Jacini, G. and Pecile, A., *Dietary Lipids and Postnatal Development*. New York: Raven Press (1973).
112. Galliard, T., *Form and Function of Phospholipids*, p. 253. G. B. Ansell, R. M. C. Dawson and J. N. Hawthorne, eds. Amsterdam: Elsevier (1973).
113. Garton, G. A., *J. Lipid Res.*, **4**, 237–254 (1963).
114. Garton, G. A., Lough, A. K. and Vioque, E., *J. Gen. Microbiol.*, **25**, 215–225 (1961).
115. Gaye, P., Haudebine, L. and Denamur, R., *Biochem. Biophys. Res. Comm.*, **51**, 637–644 (1973).
116. Glascock, R. F., Welch, V. A., Bishop, C., Davies, T., Wright, E. W. and Noble, R. C., *Biochem. J.*, **98**, 149–156 (1966).
117. Goodman, D. S., Noble, R. P. and Dell, R. B., *J. Lipid Res.*, **14**, 178–188 (1973).
118. Graziano, J. H. and Reece, R. P., *J. Dairy Sci.*, **57**, 32–35 (1974).
119. Griel, L. C. and McCarthy, R. D., *J. Dairy Sci.*, **52**, 1233–1243 (1969).
120. Griffiths, M., McIntosh, D. L. and Leckie, R. M. C., *J. Zool. Lond.*, **166**, 265–275 (1972).
121. Grove, S. N., Bracker, C. E. and Morré, D. J., *Science*, **161**, 171–173 (1968).
122. Guidotti, G., *Ann. Rev. Biochem.*, **41**, 731–752 (1972).
123. Gurr, M. I. and James, A. T., *Lipid Biochemistry*, p. 5. Ithaca, New York: Cornell University Press (1971).
124. Hajra, A. K. and Agranoff, B. W., *J. Biol. Chem.*, **243**, 3542–3543 (1968).
125. Hallgren, B. and Larsson, S., *J. Lipid Res.*, **3**, 39–43 (1962).
126. Hamilton, R. L., Havel, R. J., Kane, J. P., Blaurock, A. E. and Sata, T., *Science*, **172**, 475–478 (1971).
127. Hansen, R. P., *J. Dairy Res.*, **36**, 77–85 (1969).
128. Hansen, R. P. and Shortland, F. B., *Biochem. J.*, **52**, 207–216 (1952).
129. Hart, I. C., *J. Endocr.*, **57**, 179–180 (1973).
130. Hartman, A. M. and Dryden, L. P., *Fundamentals of Dairy Chemistry*, pp. 261–338. B. H. Webb and A. H. Johnson, eds. Westport, Connecticut: Avi Publishing Co. (1965).
131. Havel, R. J., Shore, V. G., Shore, B. and Bier, D. M., *Circ. Res.*, **27**, 595–600 (1970).
132. Hawke, J. C. and Silcock, W. R., *Biochem. J.*, **12**, 131–132 (1969).
133. Hay, J. D. and Morrison, W. R., *Biochim. Biophys. Acta*, **248**, 71–79 (1971).
134. Heald, C. W. and Saacke, R. G., *J. Dairy Sci.*, **55**, 621–628 (1972).
135. Hendler, R. W., *Physiol. Rev.*, **51**, 66–97 (1971).
136. Henson, A. F., Holdsworth, G. and Chandan, R. C., *J. Dairy Sci.*, **54**, 1752–1763 (1971).
137. Hitchcock, C. and Nichols, B. W., *Plant Lipid Biochemistry*, London and New York: Academic Press (1971).
138. Holtzman, J. L., Gram, T. E. and Gillette, J. R., *Arch. Biochem. Biophys.*, **138**, 199–207 (1970).
139. Homer, D. R. and Virtanen, A. I., *Milchwissenschaft*, **22**, 1–7 (1967).
140. Hood, L. F. and Patton, S., *J. Dairy Sci.*, **56**, 858–863 (1973).
141. Hostetler, K. Y., van den Bosch, H. and van Deenen, L. L. M., *Biochim. Biophys. Acta*, **260**, 507–513 (1972).
142. Huang, C. M. and Keenan, T. W., *J. Dairy Sci.*, **54**, 1395–1405 (1971).
143. Huang, C. M. and Keenan, T. W., *J. Dairy Sci.*, **55**, 862–864 (1972).
144. Huang, C. M. and Keenan, T. W., *Biochim. Biophys. Acta*, **274**, 246–257 (1972).
145. Huang, R. T. C., *Biochim. Biophys. Acta*, **306**, 82–84 (1973).
146. Huang, T. C. and Kuksis, A., *Lipids*, **2**, 453–460 (1967).
147. Hübscher, G., *Lipid Metabolism*, pp. 280–370, S. J. Wakil, ed. New York: Academic Press (1970).
148. Hungate, R. E., *The Rumen and Its Microbes*. New York: Academic Press (1966).
149. Hutton, J. T. and Patton, S., *J. Dairy Sci.*, **35**, 699–705 (1952).
150. Insull, W., Jr., Hirsch, J., James, A. T. and Ahrens, E. H., Jr., *J. Clin. Invest.*, **38**, 443–450 (1959).
151. Iverson, J. L., *J. Assn. Off. Anal. Chemists'*, **50**, 1118–1123 (1967).
152. Jacotot, B., Monnier, G. and Beaumont, J. L., *Clin. Chim. Acta*, **33**, 95–100 (1971).
153. James, A. T. and Martin, A. J. P., *Biochem. J.*, **63**, 144–152 (1956).
154. Jenness, R. and Patton, S., *Principles of Dairy Chemistry*. New York: John Wiley (1959).
155. Jenness, R. and Sloan, R. E., *Dairy Sci. Abstr.*, **32**, 599–612 (1970).
156. Jensen, R. G., *Progress in the Chemistry of Fats and Other Lipids*, Vol. 11, pp. 349–394. R. T. Holman, ed. Oxford: Pergamon Press (1971).
157. Jensen, R. G. *J. Amer. Oil Chemists' Soc.*, **50**, 186–192 (1973).
158. Jensen, R. G., Gander, G. W. and Sampugna, J., *J. Dairy Sci.*, **45**, 329–331 (1962).
159. Jensen, R. G., Quinn, J. G., Carpenter, D. L. and Sampugna, J., *J. Dairy Sci.* **50**, 119–126 (1967).
160. Jensen, R. G. and Sampugna, J., *J. Dairy Sci.*, **49**, 460–468 (1966).

REFERENCES

161. JENSEN, R. G., SAMPUGNA, J. and GANDER, G. W., *J. Dairy Sci.*, **44**, 1983–1988 (1961).
162. KANOH, H. and OHNO, K., *Biochim. Biophys. Acta*, **326**, 17–25 (1973).
163. KATES, M., *Techniques of Lipidology*. New York: American Elsevier (1972).
164. KATZ, I. and KEENEY, M., *J. Dairy Sci.* **49**, 962–966 (1966).
165. KATZ, I. and KEENEY, M., *Biochim. Biophys. Acta*, **44**, 102–112 (1967).
166. KAYSER, S. G. and PATTON, S., *Biochem. Biophys. Res. Comm.*, **41**, 1572–1578 (1970).
167. KEENAN, T. W., *J. Dairy Sci.*, **57**, 187–192 (1974).
168. KEENAN, T. W. and HUANG, C. M., *J. Dairy Sci.*, **55**, 1586–1596 (1972).
169. KEENAN, T. W., HUANG, C. M. and MORRÉ, D. J., *J. Dairy Sci.*, **55**, 51–57 (1972).
170. KEENAN, T. W., HUANG, C. M. and MORRÉ, D. J., *J. Dairy Sci.*, **55**, 1577–1585 (1972).
171. KEENAN, T. W., HUANG, C. M. and MORRÉ, D. J., *Biochem. Biophys. Res. Comm.*, **47**, 1277–1283 (1972).
172. KEENAN, T. W. and MORRÉ, D. J., *Biochemistry*, **9**, 19–25 (1970).
173. KEENAN, T. W. and MORRÉ, D. J., *Science*, **182**, 935–937 (1973).
174. KEENAN, T. W., MORRÉ, D. J. and CHEETHAM, R. D., *Nature*, **228**, 1105–1106 (1970).
175. KEENAN, T. W., MORRÉ, D. J. and HUANG, C. M. *Lactation: A Comprehensive Treatise*, Vol. II. B. L. Larson and V. R. Smith, eds. New York and London: Academic Press (1973).
176. KEENAN, T. W., MORRÉ, D. J., OLSON, D. E., YUNGHANS, W. N. and PATTON, S., *J. Cell Biol.*, **44**, 80–93 (1970).
177. KEENAN, T. W., OLSON, D. E. and MOLLENHAUER, H. H., *J. Dairy Sci.*, **54**, 295–299 (1971).
178. KEENAN, T. W. and PATTON, S., *Lipids*, **5**, 42–48 (1970).
179. KEENAN, T. W., SAACKE, R. G. and PATTON, S., *J. Dairy Sci.*, **53**, 1349–1352 (1970).
180. KENNEDY, E. P., *Ann. Rev. Biochem.*, **26**, 119–148 (1957).
181. KEPLER, C. R., TUCKER, W. P. and TOVE, S. B., *J. Biol. Chem.*, **246**, 2765–2771 (1971).
182. KING, N., *The Milk Fat Globule Membrane*. Furnham Royal, Bucks: Commonwealth Agricultural Bureau (1955).
183. KINSELLA, J. E., *J. Dairy Sci.*, **51**, 956 (1968).
184. KINSELLA, J. E., *J. Dairy Sci.*, **51**, 1968–1970 (1968).
185. KINSELLA, J. E., *Biochim. Biophys. Acta*, **164**, 540–549 (1968).
186. KINSELLA, J. E., *Biochim. Biophys. Acta*, **210**, 23–38 (1970).
187. KINSELLA, J. E., *Int. J. Biochem.*, **3**, 89–92 (1972).
188. KINSELLA, J. E., *Lipids*, **7**, 165–170 (1972).
189. KINSELLA, J. E., *Lipids*, **7**, 349–355 (1972).
190. KINSELLA, J. E., *Lipids*, **8**, 393–400 (1973).
191. KINSELLA, J. E. and HEALD, C. W., *J. Dairy Sci.*, **55**, 1085–1092 (1972).
192. KINSELLA, J. E. and MCCARTHY, R. D., *Biochim. Biophys. Acta*, **164**, 518–529 (1968).
193. KINSELLA, J. E., PATTON, S. and DIMICK, P. S., *J. Amer. Oil Chemists' Soc.*, **44**, 449–454 (1967).
194. KINURA, T., *J. Japan Obstet. Gynec. Soc.*, **21**, 301–308 (1969).
195. KLENK, E. and KAHLKE, W., *Z. Physiol. Chem.*, **333**, 133–139 (1963).
196. KOBYLKA, D. and CARRAWAY, K. L., *Biochim. Biophys. Acta*, **288**, 282–295 (1972).
197. KOBYLKA, D. and CARRAWAY, K. L., *Biochim. Biophys. Acta*, **307**, 133–140 (1973).
198. KON, S. K. and COWIE, A. T., eds., *Milk: The Mammary Gland and Its Secretion*, Vols. I and II. New York and London: Academic Press (1961).
199. KREIBICH, G. and SABATINI, D. D., *Fed. Proc.*, **32**, 2133–2138 (1973).
200. KUHN, N. J., *Biochem. J.*, **105**, 213–224 (1967).
201. KUHN, N. J., *Biochem. J.*, **105**, 225–231 (1967).
202. KUKSIS, A., *Progress in the Chemistry of Fats and Other Lipids*, Vol. 12, p. 82. R. T. Holman, ed. Oxford: Pergamon Press (1972).
203. KUKSIS, A. and BRECKENRIDGE, W. C., *Dairy Lipids and Lipid Metabolism*, pp. 28–98. M. F. Brink and D. Kritchevsky, eds. Westport, Connecticut: Avi Publishing Co. (1968).
204. KUKSIS, A., MARAI, L. and MYHER, J. J., *J. Amer. Oil Chemists' Soc.*, **50**, 193–201 (1973).
205. KUMAR, S., SINGH, V. N. and KEREN-PAZ, R., *Biochim. Biophys. Acta*, **98**, 221–229 (1965).
206. LACROIX, D. E., MATTINGLY, W. A., WONG, N. P. and ALFORD, J. A., *J. Amer. Dietetic Assoc.*, **62**, 275–279 (1973).
207. LANG, P. D. and INSULL, W., JR., *J. Clin. Invest.* **49**, 1479–1488 (1970).
208. LA ROSA, J. C., LEVY, R. I., HERBERT, P., LUX, S. E. and FREDERICKSON, D. S., *Biochem. Biophys. Res. Comm.*, **41**, 57–62 (1970).
209. LARSON, B. L. and SMITH, V. R., eds., *Lactation: A Comprehensive Treatise*, Vols. I, II and III. New York and London: Academic Press (1974).
210. LAURYSSENS, M., VERBEKE, R. and PETERS, G., *J. Lipid Res.*, **2**, 383–388 (1961).
211. LAWRENCE, J. G., *J. Chromat.*, **84**, 299–308 (1973).
212. LAWRENCE, R. C. and HAWKE, J. C., *Biochem. J.*, **98**, 25–29 (1966).

213. LEE, T.-C., STEPHENS, N., MOEHL, A. and SNYDER, F., *Biochim. Biophys. Acta*, **291**, 86–92 (1973).
214. LEHNINGER, A. L., *Biochemistry*. New York: Worth Publishers (1972).
215. LESKES, A., SIEKEVITZ, P. and PALADE, G. E., *J. Cell Biol.*, **49**, 264–302 (1971).
216. LEWIS, D., ed., *Digestive Physiology and Nutrition of the Ruminant*. London: Butterworth (1961).
217. LEWIS, R. W., *Lipids*, **8**, 321–323 (1973).
218. LIN, C. Y. and KUMAR, S., *J. Biol. Chem.*, **247**, 604–606 (1972).
219. LINZELL, J. L., *Nature*, **228**, 1007 (1970).
220. LINZELL, J. L., ANNISON, E. F., FAZAKERLEY, S. and LENG, R. A., *Biochem. J.*, **104**, 34–42 (1967).
221. LINZELL, J. L. and PEAKER, M., *Physiol. Rev.*, **51**, 564–597 (1971).
222. LITCHFIELD, C., *Analysis of Triglycerides*. New York and London: Academic Press (1972).
223. LOUGH, A. K., *Lipids*, **5**, 201–203 (1970).
224. LUCY, J. A., *Nature*, **227**, 815–817 (1970).
225. LUICK, J. R., *J. Dairy Sci.*, **44**, 652–657 (1961).
226. MACMAHON, B., LIN, T. M., LOWE, C. R., MIRRA, A. P., RAVNIHAR, B., SALBER, E. J., TRICHNOPOULOS, D., VALAORAS, V. G. and YUASA, S., *Bull. World Health Org.*, **42**, 185–194 (1970).
227. MAJERUS, P. W. and VAGELOS, P. R., *Advances in Lipid Research*, Vol. 5, pp. 1–33. R. Paoletti and D. Kritchevsky, eds. New York and London: Academic Press (1967).
228. MARAI, L., BRECKENRIDGE, W. C. and KUKSIS, A. *Lipids*, **4**, 562–570 (1969).
229. MARTEL, M. B., DUBOIS, P. and GOT, R., *Biochim. Biophys. Acta*, **311**, 565–575 (1973).
230. MARTEL-PRADAL, M. B. and GOT, R., *FEBS Letters*, **21**, 220–222 (1972)
231. MATA, L. J. and WYATT, R. G., *Amer. J. Clin. Nutr.*, **24**, 976–986 (1971).
232. MATTSON, F. H., ERICKSON, B. A. and KLIGMAN, A. M., *Amer. J. Clin. Nutr.*, **25**, 589–594 (1972).
233. MCBRIDE, O. W. and KORN, E. D., *J. Lipid Res.*, **4**, 17–20 (1963).
234. MCBRIDE, O. W. and KORN, E. D., *J. Lipid Res.*, **5**, 442–447 (1964).
235. MCBRIDE, O. W. and KORN, E. D., *J. Lipid Res.*, **5**, 448–452 (1964).
236. MCCARTHY, R. D., GHIARDI, F. L. A. and PATTON, S., *Biochim. Biophys. Acta*, **98**, 216–217 (1965).
237. MCCARTHY, R. D. and PATTON, S., *Biochim. Biophys. Acta*, **70**, 102–103 (1963).
238. MCCARTHY, R. D. and PATTON, S., *Nature*, **202**, 347–349 (1964).
239. MCCARTHY, S. and SMITH, G. H., *Biochim. Biophys. Acta*, **260**, 185–196 (1972).
240. MCKENZIE, H. A., ed., *Milk Proteins: Chemistry and Molecular Biology*, Vol. II. New York and London: Academic Press (1971).
241. MENDELSON, C. E. and SCOW, R. O., *Amer. J. Physiol.*, **223**, 1418–1423 (1972).
242. MILLS, E. S. and TOPPER, Y. J., *J. Cell Biol.*, **44**, 310–328 (1970).
243. MORRÉ, D. J., MOLLENHAUER, H. H. and BRACKER, C. E. *Results and Problems in Cell Differentiation*, Vol. 2, pp. 82–126. J. Reinert and H. Ursprung, eds. Berlin, Heidelberg, New York: Springer-Verlag (1971).
244. MORRISON, W. R., *Biochim. Biophys. Acta*, **176**, 537–546 (1969).
245. MORRISON, W. R., *Topics in Lipid Chemistry*, Vol. 1, pp. 52–95. F. D. Gunstone, ed. New York: John Wiley (1970).
246. MORRISON, W. R., *FEBS Letters*, **19**, 63–64 (1971).
247. MORRISON, W. R., *Biochim. Biophys. Acta*, **316**, 98–107 (1973).
248. MORRISON, W. R. and HAY, J. D., *Biochim. Biophys. Acta*, **202**, 460–467 (1970).
249. MUKHERJEE, A. S., WASHBURN, L. L. and MANERJEE, M. R., *Nature*, **246**, 159–160 (1973).
250. MULDER, H. and ZUIDHOF, T. A., *Neth. Milk Dairy J.*, **12**, 173–179 (1958).
251. MURATA, T. and TAKAHASHI, S., *Anal. Chem.*, **45**, 1816–1823 (1973).
252. MUTO, Y., SMITH, F. R. and GOODMAN, D. S., *J. Lipid Res.*, **14**, 525–532 (1973).
253. NELSON, G. J., *Blood Lipids and Lipoproteins: Quantitation, Composition and Metabolism*. New York: Wiley Interscience (1972).
254. NESTEL, P. J., HAVENSTEIN, N., WHYTE, H. M., SCOTT, T. J. and COOK, L. J., *New Engl. J. Med.*, **288** (8), 379–382 (1973).
255. NEWMAN, R. A. and HARRISON, R., *Biochim. Biophys. Acta*, **298**, 798–809 (1973).
256. NOVIKOFF, A. B., ROHEIM, P. S. and QUINTANA, N., *Lab. Invest.*, **15**, 27–49 (1966)
257. NUTTER, L. J. and PRIVETT, O. S., *J. Dairy Sci.*, **50**, 298–304 (1967).
258. NUTTER, L. J. and PRIVETT, O. S., *J. Dairy Sci.*, **50**, 1194–1199 (1967).
259. OCKNER, R. F., HUGHES, F. B. and ISSELBACHER, K. J., *J. Clin. Invest.*, **48**, 2079–2088 (1969).
260. OCKNER, R. F., MANNING, J. A., POPPENHAUSEN, R. B. and HO, W. K. L., *Science*, **177**, 56–58 (1972).
261. OKA, T. and TOPPER, Y. J., *J. Biol. Chem.*, **246**, 7701–7707 (1971).
262. OKA, T. and TOPPER, Y. J., *Nature New Biology*, **239**, 216–217 (1972).
263. ORCI, L., LE MARCHAND, Y., SINGH, A., ASSIMACOPOULOS-JEANNET, F., ROUILLER, C. and JEANRENAUD, B., *Nature*, **244**, 30–32 (1973).
264. PARKS, O. W., KEENEY, M. and SCHWARTZ D. P., *J. Dairy Sci.*, **44**, 1940–1943 (1961).
265. PARSONS, J. G. and PATTON, S., *J. Lipid Res.*, **8**, 696–698 (1967).

REFERENCES

266. PATTON, R. A., MCCARTHY, R. D. and GRIEL, L. C., *J. Dairy Sci.*, **53**, 460–465 (1970).
267. PATTON, S., *J. Theoret. Biol.*, **29**, 489–491 (1970).
268. PATTON, S., *Nature*, **228**, 97 (1970).
269. PATTON, S., *J. Amer. Oil Chemists' Soc.*, **50**, 178–185 (1973).
270. PATTON, S. and BENSON, A. A., *Biochim. Biophys. Acta*, **125**, 22–32 (1966).
271. PATTON, S. DURDAN, A. and MCCARTHY, R. D., *J. Dairy Sci.*, **47**, 489–495 (1964).
272. PATTON, S. and FOWKES, F. M., *J. Theoret. Biol.*, **15**, 274–281 (1967).
273. PATTON, S. and HOOD, L. F., *Lactogenesis: The Initiation of Milk Secretion at Parturition*, pp. 121–129. M. Reynolds and S. J. Folley, eds. Philadelphia: University of Pennsylvania Press (1969).
274. PATTON, S., HOOD, L. F. and PATTON, J. S., *J. Lipid Res.*, **10**, 260–266 (1969).
275. PATTON, S. and KEENAN, T. W., *Lipids*, **6**, 58–62 (1971).
276. PATTON, S. and KESLER, E. M., *Science*, **156**, 1365–1366 (1967).
277. PATTON, S. and KESLER, E. M., *J. Dairy Sci.*, **50**, 1505–1508 (1967).
278. PATTON, S. and MCCARTHY, R. D., *J. Dairy Sci.*, **46**, 396–400 (1963).
279. PATTON, S. and MCCARTHY, R. D., *J. Dairy Sci.*, **46**, 916–921 (1963).
280. PATTON, S. and MCCARTHY, R. D., *Nature*, **209**, 616–617 (1966).
281. PATTON, S., MCCARTHY, R. D. and DIMICK. P. S., *J. Dairy Sci.*, **48**, 1389–1391 (1965).
282. PATTON, S., MCCARTHY, R. D., EVANS, L. and LYNN, T. R., *J. Dairy Sci.*, **43**, 1187–1195 (1960).
283. PATTON, S., MCCARTHY, R. D., PLANTZ, P. E. and LEE, R .F., *Nature New Biology*, **241**, 241–242 (1973).
284. PATTON, S., MUMMA, R. O. and MCCARTHY, R. D., Abstracts of Papers (No. 103), 40th Fall Meeting, Am. Oil Chemists' Soc., Phila., Pa. (1966).
285. PATTON, S., PLANTZ, P. E. and THOELE, C. A., *J. Dairy Sci.*, **56**, 1473–1476 (1973).
286. PATTON, S. and TRAMS, E. G., *FEBS Letters*, **14**, 230–232 (1971).
287. PEEREBOOM, J. W. C., *Fette Seifen Anstrichm.*, **71**, 314–322 (1969).
288. PELC, S. and FELL, H. D., *Exp. Cell Res.*, **19**, 99–113 (1960).
289. PHILLIPSON, A. T., ed., *Physiology of Digestion and Metabolism in the Ruminant*. Newcastle upon Tyne: Oriel Press (1970).
290. PITAS, R. E., SAMPUGNA, J. and JENSEN, R. G., *J. Dairy Sci.*, **50**, 1332–1336 (1967).
291. PLANTZ, P. E. and PATTON, S., *Biochim. Biophys. Acta*, **291**, 51–60 (1973).
292. PLANTZ, P. E., PATTON, S. and KEENAN, T. W., *J. Dairy Sci.*, **56**, 978–983 (1973).
293. PLOWMAN, R. D., BITMAN, J., GORDON, C. H., DRYDEN, L. P., GORRING, H. K., WRENN, T. R., EDMONDSON, L. F., YONCOSKIE, R. A. and DOUGLAS, F. W., JR., *J. Dairy Sci.*, **55**, 204–207 (1972).
294. POLHEIM, D., DAVID, J. S. K., SCHULTZ, F. M., WYLIE, M. B. and JOHNSTON, J. M. *J. Lipid Res.*, **14**, 415–421 (1973).
295. POLIS, B. D., SHMUKLER, H. W. and CUSTER, J. H., *J. Biol. Chem.*, **187**, 349–354 (1950).
296. POPJACK, G., FRENCH, T. H., HUNTER, G. D. and MARTIN, A. J. P., *Biochem. J.*, **48**, 612–618 (1951).
297. PORTMAN, O. W., *Advances in Lipid Research*, Vol. 8, pp. 41–114. R. Paoletti and D. Kritchevsky, eds. New York and London: Academic Press (1970).
298. PORTMAN, O. W. and ALEXANDER, M., *Biochim. Biophys. Acta*, **260**, 460–474 (1972).
299. PRENTICE, J. H., *Dairy Sci. Abstr.*, **31**, 353–356 (1969).
300. PYNADATH, T. I. and KUMAR, S., *Biochim. Biophys. Acta*, **84**, 251–263 (1964).
301. RAPHAEL, B. C., DIMICK, P. S. and PUPPIONE, D. L., *J. Dairy Sci.*, **56**, 1025–1032 (1973).
302. RAPHAEL, B. C., DIMICK, P. S. and PUPPIONE, D. L., *J. Dairy Sci.*, **56**, 1411–1414 (1973).
303. REISER, R., *Fed. Proc.*, **10**, 236 (1951).
304. REISER, R. and SIDELMAN, Z., *J. Nutr.*, **102**, 1009–1016 (1972).
305. REYNOLDS, J. A., *Fed. Proc.*, **32**, 2034–2038 (1973).
306. REYNOLDS, M. and FOLLEY, S. J., eds., *Lactogenesis: The Initiation of Milk Secretion at Parturition*. Philadelphia: University of Pennyslvania Press (1969).
307. ROBINSON, D. S., *J. Lipid Res.*, **4**, 21–23 (1963).
308. RISTOW, R. and WERNER, H., *Fette Seifen Anstrichm.*, **70**, 273–288 (1968).
309. ROSEMAN, S., *Chem. Phys. Lipids*, **5**, 270–297 (1970).
310. ROSENFELD, I. S. and TOVE, S. B., *J. Biol. Chem.*, **246**, 5025–5030 (1971).
311. ROTHMAN, J. E. and ENGLEMAN, D. M., *Nature New Biology*, **237**, 42–44 (1972).
312. ROUSER, G. and SOLOMAN, R. D., *Lipids*, **4**, 232–234 (1969).
313. RUSSFIELD, A. B., *Tumors of Endocrine Glands and Secondary Sex Organs*, pp. 87–91. D. J Taylor, ed. Washington, D. C.: Public Health Service Publication No. 1332 (1966).
314. RYHAGE, B., *J. Dairy Res.*, **34**, 115–121 (1967).
315. SAACKE, R. G. and HEALD, C. W., *Lactation: A Comprehensive Treatise*, Vol. II. B. L. Larson and V. R. Smith, eds. New York and London: Academic Press (1974).
316. SAMPUGNA, J., QUINN, J. G., PITAS, R. E., CARPENTER, D. L. and JENSEN, R.G., *Lipids*, **2**, 397–402 (1967).

317. Samuel, P. and Lieberman, S., *J. Lipid Res.*, **14**, 189–196 (1973).
318. Scanu, A. M., *Biochim. Biophys. Acta*, **265**, 471–508 (1972).
319. Schams, D., Reinhardt, V. and Karg, H., *Milchwissenschaft*, **28**, 409–418 (1973).
320. Schoefl, G. I. and French, J. E., *Proc. Roy. Soc. B*, **169**, 153–165 (1968).
321. Schotz, M. C. and Garfinkel, A. S., *Biochim. Biophys. Acta*, **270**, 472–478 (1972).
322. Schwartz, D. P. Paper presented at 46th Fall Meeting, Amer. Oil Chemists' Soc., Abstract No. 96, *J. Amer. Oil Chemists' Soc.*, **49**, 312A (1972).
323. Scott, T. W., Cook, L. J., Ferguson, K. A., McDonald, I. W., Buchanan, R. A. and Loftus Hills, G., *Aust. J. Sci.*, **32**, 291–293 (1970).
324. Scott, T. W., Cook, L. J. and Mills, S. C., *J. Amer. Oil Chemists' Soc.*, **48**, 358–364 (1971).
325. Scow, R. O., Hamosh, M., Blanchette-Mackie, E. J. and Evans, A. J., *Lipids*, **7**, 497–505 (1972).
326. Searcy, R. L., Bergquist, L. M. and Jung, R. C., *J. Lipid Res.*, **4**, 349–351 (1960).
327. Senior, J. R., *J. Lipid Res.*, **5**, 495–512 (1964).
328. Shahani, K. M., *J. Dairy Sci.*, **49**, 907–920 (1966).
329. Shehata, A. A. Y. and deMan, J. M., *Can. Inst. Food Technol. J.*, **4**, 38–44 (1971).
330. Shehata, A. A. Y., deMan, J. M. and Alexander, J. C., *Can. Inst. Food Technol. J.*, **3**, 85–89 (1970).
331. Shehata, A. A. Y., deMan, J. M. and Alexander, J. C., *Can. Inst. Food Technol. J.*, **4**, 61–67 (1971).
332. Shehata, A. A. Y., deMan, J. M. and Alexander, J. C., *Can. Inst. Food Technol. J.*, **5**, 13–21 (1972).
333. Sherbon, J. W. and Dolby, R. M., *J. Dairy Res.*, **39**, 325–333 (1972).
334. Silcock, W. R. and Patton, S., *J. Cell. Physiol.*, **79**, 151–154 (1972).
335. Singer, S. J. and Nicholson, G. L., *Science*, **175**, 720–731 (1972).
336. Slomiany, B. L. and Horowitz, M. I., *Biochim. Biophys. Acta*, **218**, 278–287 (1970).
337. Smith, C. R., Jr., *Progress in the Chemistry of Fats and Other Lipids*, Vol. 11, p. 139. R. T. Holman, ed. Oxford: Pergamon Press (1970).
338. Smith, L. M., ed., *Symposium: Milk Lipids. J. Amer. Oil Chemists' Soc.*, **50**, 175–201 (1973).
339. Smith, S., *Arch. Biochem. Biophys.*, **156**, 751–758 (1973).
340. Smith, S. and Abraham, S., *J. Biol. Chem.*, **246**, 6428–6435 (1971).
341. Snipes, M. B. and Lengemann, F. W., *J. Dairy Sci.*, **55**, 1783–1786 (1972).
342. Solyom, A. and Trams, E. G., *Enzyme*, **13**, 329 372 (1972).
343. Stein, O. and Stein, Y., *J. Cell Biol.*, **33**, 319–339 (1967).
344. Stein, O. and Stein, Y., *J. Cell Biol.*, **34**, 251–263 (1967).
345. Stein, O. and Stein, Y., *Biochim. Biophys. Acta*, **306**, 142–147 (1973).
346. Steinberg, D., Herndon, J. H., Jr., Uhlendorf, B. W., Mize, C. E., Avigan, J. and Milne, G. W. A., *Science*, **156**, 1740–1742 (1967).
347. Stewart, P. S., Ph.D. Thesis. University of Guelph, Canada (1970).
348. Stewart, P. S., Puppione, D. L. and Patton, S., *Z. Zellforsch.*, **123**, 161–167 (1972).
349. Storry, J. E., *J. Dairy Res.*, **37**, 139–164 (1970).
350. Strocchi, A. and Holman, R. T., *Riv. Ital. Sostanze Grasse*, **48**, 617–622 (1971).
351. Strong, C., Dils, R. and Forsyth, I. A., *J. Endocr.*, **51**, xxxii–xxxiii (1971).
352. Swenson, P. E., Dimick, P. S. and Walker, N. J., *J. Dairy Sci.*, **56**, 1337–1339 (1973).
353. Taylor, C. B., Mickelson, B., Anderson, J. A. and Forman, D. Y., *Arch. Pathol.*, **81**, 213–231 (1966).
354. Timmen, H. and Dimick, P. S., *J. Dairy Sci.*, **55**, 919–925 (1972).
355. Traurig, H. H., *Anat. Record*, **157**, 489–503 (1967).
356. Turkington, R. W., *Biochem. Biophys. Res. Comm.*, **41**, 1362–1367 (1970).
357. Turkington, R. W., Brew, K., Vanaman, T. C. and Hill, R. L., *J. Biol. Chem.*, **243**, 3382–3387 (1968).
358. Turkington, R. W. and Hill, R. L., *Science*, **163**, 1458–1460 (1969).
359. Vagelos, P. R., Majerus, P. W., Alberts, A. W., Larrabee, A. R. and Ailhaud, G. P., *Fed. Proc.*, **35**, 1485–1494 (1966).
360. Vaidya, A., *Science*, **180**, 776–779 (1973).
361. VanDeenan, L. L. M., *Progress in the Chemistry of Fats and Other Lipids*, Vol. 8, pp. 1–127. R. T. Holman, ed. Oxford: Pergamon Press (1965).
362. Van der Wel, H. and de Jong, K., *Fette Seifen Anstrichm.*, **67**, 279–281 (1969).
363. Van Golde, L. M. G., Fleischer, B. and Fleischer, S., *Biochim. Biophys. Acta*, **249**, 318–330 (1971).
364. Virtanen, A. I., *Science*, **153**, 1603–1614 (1966).
365. Visser, A. S., de Haas, W. R. E., Knox, C. and Prop, F. J. A., *Exptl. Cell Res.*, **73**, 516–519 (1972).

366. VIVIANI, R., *Advances in Lipid Research*, Vol. 8, pp. 268–346. R. Paoletti and D. Kritchevsky, eds. New York: Academic Press (1970).
367. WAKIL, S. J., *J. Lipid Res.*, **2**, 1–24 (1961).
368. WALKER, N. J., PATTON, S. and DIMICK, P. S., *Biochim. Biophys. Acta*, **152**, 445–453 (1968).
369. WEBB, B. H. and JOHNSON, A. H., eds., *Fundamentals of Dairy Chemistry*. Westport, Connecticut: Avi Publishing Co. (1965).
370. WEIHRAUCH, J. L., BREWINGTON, C. R. and SCHWARTZ, D. P., *Lipids*, **9**, 883–890 (1974).
371. WEISS, S. B., KENNEDY, E. P. and KIYASU, J. Y., *J. Biol. Chem.*, **235**, 40–43 (1960).
372. WELLINGS, S. R., GRUNBAUM, B. W. and DEOME, K. B., *J. Nat. Cancer Inst.*, **25**, 423–437 (1960).
373. WEST, C. E., BICKERSTAFFE, R., ANNISON, E. F., and LINZELL, J. L., *Biochem. J.*, **126**, 477–490 (1972).
374. WHITE, R. F., EATON, H. D. and PATTON, S., *J. Dairy Sci.*, **37**, 147–155 (1954).
375. WIDNELL, C. C. and UNKELESS, J. C., *Proc. Nat. Acad. Sci.*, **61**, 1050–1059 (1968).
376. WILSON, J. D. and LINDSEY, C. A., Jr., *J. Clin. Invest.*, **44**, 1805–1814 (1965).
377. WINDMUELLER, H. G., HERBERT, P. N. and LEVY, R. I., *J. Lipid Res.*, **14**, 215–223 (1973).
378. WOODING, F. B. P., *J. Ultrastruct. Res.*, **37**, 388–400 (1971).
379. WOODING, F. B. P., *J. Cell Sci.*, **9**, 805–821 (1971).
380. WOODING, F. B. P., *Experientia*, **28**, 1077–1079 (1972).
381. WOODING, F. B. P., PEAKER, M. and LINZELL, J. L., *Nature*, **226**, 762–764 (1970).
382. WRIGHT, J. D. and GREEN, C., *Biochem. J.*, **123**, 837–844 (1971).
383. WUNDERLICH, F., MULLER, R. and SPETH, V., *Science*, **182**, 1136–1138 (1973).
384. WYNDER, E. L., *Cancer*, **24**, 1235–1240 (1969).
385. YANG, S. F., FREER, S. and BENSON, A. A., *J. Biol. Chem.*, **242**, 477–484 (1967).
386. ZILVERSMIT, D. B., *J. Clin. Invest.*, **44**, 1610–1622 (1965).
387. ZILVERSMIT, D. B., *Fed. Proc.*, **26**, 1599–1605 (1967).

ADDENDUM

In the year or so since writing for the first edition of this work was completed, several hundred publications dealing directly with mammary tissue or milk have come to the authors' attention. As a guide for additional reading and to update areas of research some of these papers and books are listed below.

1. Hormones, regulators and differentiation

(a) Reviews

CONVEY, E. M. Serum hormone concentration in ruminants during mammary growth, lactogenesis and lactation: a review. *J. Dairy Sci.*, **57**, 905–917 (1974).
HEALD, C. W. Hormonal effects on mammary cytology. *J. Dairy Sci.*, **57**, 917–925 (1974).

(b) Prolactin (see also lipoprotein lipase and breast cancer)

CHOMCZYNSKI, P. and TOPPER, Y. J. A direct effect of prolactin and placental lactogen on mammary epithelial nuclei. *Biochem. Biophys. Res. Comm.*, **60**, 56–63 (1974).
HART, I. C. Concentration of prolactin in serial blood samples from goats before, during and after milking throughout lactation. *J. Endocr.*, **64**, 305–312 (1975).
HART, I. C. Seasonal factors affecting the release of prolactin in goats in response to milking. *J. Endocr.*, **64**, 313–322 (1975).
MCMURTRY, J. P., MALVEN, P. V., ARAVE, C. W., ERB, R. E. and HARRINGTON, R. B. Environmental and lactational variables affecting prolactin concentrations in bovine milk. *J. Dairy Sci.*, **58**, 181–189 (1975).
SHIU, R. P. C. and FRIESEN, H. G. Solubilization and purification of a prolactin receptor from the rabbit mammary gland. *J. Biol. Chem.*, **249**, 7902–7911 (1974).
TYSON, J. E., KHOJANDI, M., HUTH, J. and ANDREASSEN, B. The influence of prolactin on human lactation. *J. Clin. Endocrinol. Metab.*, **40**, 764–773 (1975).

(c) Spermidine

OKA, T. and PERRY, J. W. Spermidine as a possible mediator of glucocorticoid effect on milk protein synthesis in mouse mammary epithelium *in vitro*. *J. Biol. Chem.*, **249**, 7647–7652 (1974).
SANGUANSERMSRI, J., GYORGY, P. and ZILLIKEN, F. Polyamines in human and cow's milk. *Am. J. Clin. Nutr.*, **27**, 859–865 (1975).

(d) Cyclic AMP

LOIZZI, R. F., DE PONT, J. J. H. H. M. and BONTING, S. L. Inhibition by cyclic AMP of lactose production in lactating guinea pig mammary gland slices. *Biochim. Biophys. Acta*, **392**, 20–25 (1975).
LOUIS, S. L. and BALDWIN, R. L. Changes in the cyclic 3′, 5′-adenosine monophosphate system of rat mammary gland during lactation cycle. *J. Dairy Sci.*, **58**, 861–869 (1975).
SAPAG-HAGAR, M. and GREENBAUM, A. L. Adenosine 3′, 5′-monophosphate and hormone interrelationships in the mammary gland of the rat during pregnancy and lactation. *Eu. J. Biochem.*, **47**, 303–312 (1974).

(e) Calcitonin

GAREL, J. M., CARE, A. D. and BARLET, J. P. A radio-immunoassay for ovine calcitonin: an evaluation of calcitonin secretion during gestation, lactation and foetal life. *J. Endocr.*, **62**, 497–509 (1974).

(f) Prostaglandins

RILLEMA, J. A. Possible role of prostaglandin $F_{2\alpha}$ in mediating effect of prolactin and RNA synthesis in mammary gland explants of mice. *Nature*, **253**, 466–467 (1975).

(g) Progesterone

ASSAIRI, L. DELOUIS. C., GAYE, P., HOUDEBINE, L.-M., OLLIVIER-BOUSQUET, M. and DENAMUR, R. Inhibition by progesterone of the lactogenic effect of prolactin in the pseudopregnant rabbit. *Biochem. J.*, **144**, 245–252 (1974).

2. The human mammary gland

(a) Ultrastructure

OZZELLO, L. Ultrastructure of the human mammary gland. *Path. Ann.*, **6**, 1–59 (1971).
RUSSO, J., FURMASKI, P. and RICH, M. A. An ultrastructural study of normal human mammary epithelial cells in culture. *Am. J. Anat.*, **142**, 221–232 (1975).
TOBON, H. and SALAZAR, H. Ultrastructure of the human mammary gland. I. Development of the fetal gland throughout gestation. *J. Clin. Endocrinol. Metab.*, **39**, 443–456 (1974). Post-partum lactogenesis. *ibid.*, **40**, 834–844 (1975).
WAUGH, D. and VAN DER HOEVEN, E. Fine structure of the human adult female breast. *Lab. Invest.* **11**, 220–228 (1962).

(b) Breast function and care

VORHERR, H. *The Breast*. New York, San Francisco and London: Academic Press (1974).
ROTHENBERG, R. E. *Breast Care*. New York: Crown Publishers (1975).

3. Breast cancer

MARX, J. L. Breast cancer research: problems and progress. *Science*, **184**, 1162–1164 (1974).
MINTON, J. P. Prolactin and human breast cancer. *Am. J. Surg.*, **128**, 628–630 (1974).
MOORE, D. H. and CHARNEY, J. Breast cancer: etiology and possible prevention. *Amer. Sci.*, **63**, 160–168 (1975).

4. Membranes

(a) General

SINGER, S. J. The molecular organization of membranes. *Ann. Rev. Biochem.*, **43**, 805–833 (1974).

(b) Sidedness

DePIERRE, J. W. and KARNOVSKY, M. L. Ecto enzymes of the guinea pig polymorphonuclear leucocyte. I. Evidence for an ecto-adenosine monophosphatase, -adenosine triphosphatase and -*p*-nitrophenyl phosphatase. *J. Biol. Chem.*, **249**, 7111–7120 (1974); *Ibid.* II. Properties and suitability as markers for the plasma membrane, pp.7121–7129.

TRAMS, E. G. and LAUTER, C. J. On the sidedness of plasma membrane enzymes. *Biochim. Biophys. Acta*, **345**, 180–197 (1974).

TSAI, K.-H. and LEONARD, J. Asymmetry of influenza virus membrane bilayer demonstrated with phospholipase C. *Nature*, **253**, 554–555 (1974).

(c) The milk fat globule membrane

CARLBERG-BACQ, C.-M., FRANCOIS, C., GOSSELIN, L., OSTERRIETH, P. M. and RENTIER-DELRUE, F. Lipid and protein composition of the mammary tumor virus and the milk fat globule membrane isolated from the milk of infected mice. *Biochem. Soc. Trans.*, **3**, 296–299 (1975).

HARRISON, R., HIGGINBOTHAM, J. D. and NEWMAN, R. Sialoglycopeptides from bovine milk fat globule membrane. *Biochim. Biophys. Acta*, **389**, 449–463 (1975).

MANGINO, M. E. and BRUNNER, J. R. Molecular weight profile of fat globule membrane proteins. *J. Dairy Sci.*, **58**, 313–318 (1975).

MATHER, H I. and KEENAN, T. W. Studies on the structure of milk fat globule membrane. *J. Membrane Biol.*, **21**, 65–85 (1975).

MONIS, B., ROVASIO, R. A. and VALENTICH, M. A. Ultra-structural characterization by ruthenium red of the surface of the milk fat globule membrane of human and rat milk with data on carbohydrates of fractions of rat milk. *Cell Tiss. Res.*, **157**, 17–24 (1975).

PATTON, S. and KEENAN, T. W. The milk fat globule membrane *Biochim. Biophys. Acta*, **415**, 273–309 (1975).

WOODING, F. B. P. Milk fat globule membrane material in skim milk. *J. Dairy Res.*, **41**, 331–337 (1974).

5. Functioning of cell organelles

(a) Microtubules, colchicine and suppression of lactation

PATTON, S. Reversible suppression of lactation by colchicine. *FEBS Letters*, **48**, 85–87 (1974).

SANDBORN, E., KOEN, P. F., McNABB, J. D. and MOORE, G. Cytoplasmic microtubules in mammalian cells. *J. Ultrastructure Research*, **11**, 123–138 (1964).

WEISENBERGER, R. C. Microtubule formation *in vitro* in solutions containing low calcium concentration. *Science*, **177**, 1104–1105 (1972).

(b) The Golgi apparatus

(b) The Golgi apparatus

BAUMRUCKER, C. R. and KEENAN, T. W. Membranes of mammary gland. X. Adenosine triphosphate-dependent calcium accumulation by Golgi apparatus rich fractions of bovine mammary gland. *Exp. Cell Res.*, **90**, 253–260 (1975).

6. Ions and ion transport
(see also 5b)

LINZELL, J. L. and PEAKER, M. Changes in colostrum composition and in the permeability of the mammary epithelium at about the time of parturition in the goat. *J. Physiol.*, **243**, 129–151 (1974).

PEAKER, M. Recent advances in the study of monovalent ion movements across the mammary epithelium: relation to onset of lactation. *J. Dairy Sci.*, **58**, 1042–1047 (1975).

VREESWIJK, J. H. A., DE PONT, J. J. H. H. M. and BONTING, S. L. Na-K ATPase activity and intracellular ion concentrations in the lactating guinea pig mammary gland. *Pflügers Arch.*, **356**, 347–357 (1975).

VREESWIJK, J. H. A., DE PONT, J. J. H. H. M. and BONTING, S. L. (1975) Absence of Na+, K+-ATPAse involvement in lactose production by lactating guinea pig mammary gland. *Biochim. Biophys. Acta*, **392**, 12–19 (1975).

7. Lactose biosynthesis

BREW, K. and HILL, R. L. Lactose biosynthesis. *Rev. Physiol. Biochem. Pharmac.*, **72**, 105–158 (1975).
KUHN, N. J. and WHITE, A. The topography of lactose synthesis. *Biochem. J.*, **148**, 77–84 (1975).

8. Lipoprotein lipase

FALCONER, I. R. and FIDDLER, T. J. Effects of intraductal administration of prolactin, actinomycin D and cycloheximide on lipoprotein lipase activity in the mammary glands of pseudo-pregnant rabbits. *Biochim. Biophys. Acta*, **218**, 508–514 (1970).
HERNELL, O. and OLIVECRONA, T. Human milk lipases. I. Serum-stimulated lipase. *J. Lipid Res.*, **15**, 367–374 (1974).
ZINDER, O., HAMOSH, M., FLECK, T. R. C. and SCOW, R. O. Effect of prolactin on lipoprotein lipase in mammary gland and adipose tissue of rats. *Am. J. Physiol.*, **226**, 744–748 (1974).

9. Lipid metabolism

(a) Biosynthesis and structure of milk triglycerides

BARBANO, D. M. and SHERBON, J. W. Stereospecific analysis of high melting triglycerides of bovine milk fat and their biosynthetic origin. *J. Dairy Sci.*, **58**, 1–8 (1975).
CHRISTIE, W. W. Biosynthesis of triglycerides in freshly secreted milk from goats. *Lipids*, **9**, 876–882 (1974).
MCCARTHY, R. D. and COCCODRILLI, G. D., Jr. Structure and synthesis of milk fat. XI. Effect of heparin on paths of incorporation of glucose and palmitic acid into milk fat. *J. Dairy Sci.*, **58**, 164–168 (1975).
PATTON, S. Detection of rapidly labeled phosphatidic acid in lactating mammary gland of the intact rat. *J. Dairy Sci.*, **58**, 560–563 (1975).

(b) Depressed milk fat

JENNY, B. F., POLAN, C. E. and THYE, F. W. Effects of high grain feeding and stage of lactation on serum insulin, glucose and milk fat percentage in lactating cows. *J. Nutr.*, **104**, 379–385 (1974).

(c) Origin and chain length of milk triglyceride fatty acids

GLASCOCK, R. F. and WELCH, V. A. Contribution of the fatty acids of three low density serum lipoproteins to bovine milk fat. *J. Dairy Sci.*, **57**, 1364–1370 (1974).
GROSS, M. J. and KINSELLA, J. E. Properties of palmityl-CoA: 1-α-glycerolphosphate acyl transferase from bovine mammary microsomes. *Lipids*, **9**, 905–912 (1974).
KNUDSEN, J. and DILS, R. Partial purification from rabbit mammary gland of a factor which controls the chain length of fatty acids synthesized. *Biochem. Biophys. Res. Comm.*, **63**, 780–785 (1975).
SMITH, G. H., MCCARTHY, S. and ROOK, J. A. F. Synthesis of milk fat from β-hydroxybutyrate and acetate in lactating goats. *J. Dairy Res.*, **41**, 175–191 (1974).
SWENSON, P. E. and DIMICK, P. S. Oxidation of medium chain fatty acids by the ruminant mammary gland. *J. Dairy Sci.*, **57**, 290–295 (1974).

(d) Cholesterol

BERNSTEIN, B. A., RICHARDSON, T. and AMUNDSON, C. H. Inhibition of cholesterol biosynthesis by bovine milk, cultured buttermilk and orotic acid. *J. Dairy Sci.*, **58**, 790 (1975).
FRIEDMAN, G. and GOLDBERG, S. J. Concurrent and subsequent serum cholesterols of breast- and formula-fed infants. *Am. J. Clin. Nutr.*, **28**, 42–45 (1975).
RAPHAEL, B. C., PATTON, S. and MCCARTHY, R. D. Transport of dietary cholesterol into blood and milk of the goat. *J. Dairy Sci.*, **58**, 971–976 (1975).

(e) Phosphatidylcholine as a precursor of sphingomyelin

DIRINGER, H. and KOCH, M. A. Biosynthesis of sphingomyelin: transfer of phosphorylcholine from phosphatidylcholine to erythro-ceramide in a cell-free system. *Z. Physiol. Chem. Hoppe Seyler's*, **354**, 1661–1665 (1973).

ULMAN, M. D. and RADIN, N. S. The enzymatic formation of sphingomyelin from ceramide and lecithin in mouse liver. *J. Biol. Chem.*, **249**, 1506–1512 (1974).

(f) Alveoli (acini) and fat cells

ELIAS, J. J., PITELKA, D. R. and ARMSTRONG, R. C. Changes in fat cell morphology during lactation in the mouse. *Anat. Rec.*, **177**, 533–548 (1973).

KATZ, J., WALS, P. A. and VAN DE VELDE, R. L. Lipogenesis by acini from mammary gland of lactating rats. *J. Biol. Chem.*, **249**, 7348–7357 (1974).

10. *Milk lipid composition*

BREWINGTON, C. R., PARKS, O. W. and SCHWARTZ, D. P. Conjugated compounds (glucoronides and sulfates of fatty acids) in cow's milk. II. *J. Agr. Food Chem.*, **22**, 293–294 (1974).

DARLING, J. A. B., LAING, A. H. and HARKNESS, R. A. Steroids in cow's milk. *J. Endocr.*, **62**, 291–297 (1974).

FEELEY, R. M., CRINER, P. E. and SLOVER, H. T. Major fatty acids and proximate composition of dairy products. *J. Am. Diet. Assn.*, **66**, 140–145 (1975).

FLANAGAN, V. P., FERRETTI, A., SCHWARTZ, D. P. and RUTH, J. M. Steroid ketones and isoprenoid alcohols in dairy products. *J. Lipid Res.*, **16**, 97–101 (1975).

HALLGREN, B., NIKLASSON, A., STALLBERG, G. and THORIN, H. Alkyl- and 2- methoxyalkylglycerols in human, cow's and sheep's milks. *Acta Chem. Scand.*, **2813**, 1029–1034 (1974).

KEENAN, T. W. Composition and synthesis of gangliosides in mammary gland and milk of the bovine. *Biochim. Biophys. Acta*, **337**, 255–270 (1974).

POSATI, L. P., KINSELLA, J. E. and WATTS, B. K. Comprehensive evaluation of fatty acids in foods. I. Dairy products. *J. Am. Diet. Assn.*, **66**, 482–488 (1975).

URBACH, G. and STARK, W. The C-20 and other hydrocarbons of butterfat. *J. Agr. Food Chem.*, **23**, 20–24 (1975).

11. *Chemistry and technology of milk*

MULDER, H. and WALSTRA, P. *The Milk Fat Globule*. Farnham Royal, Bucks, England: Commonwealth Agricultural Bureau (1974).

WEBB, B. H., JOHNSON, A. H. and ALFORD, J. A. (eds.) *Fundamentals of Dairy Chemistry*. 2nd ed. Westport, Connecticut: AVI Publishing Co. (1974).

INDEX

Acetate metabolism 10, 12, 53, 56
Acetyl CoA carboxylase 54
Acyl carrier protein 54
Acyl transferase 37, 58
Adipose tissue 3, 11, 20, 22–24, 29
Aging 2
Aldehydes, bound in glycerides 84
Alveolus 22–25
AMP, cyclic 34
Atherosclerosis 14, 20, 34, 67, 68, 94
ATP 30, 75
ATPase 25, 35, 49–51

Bacteria, rumen 11, 13
Bases, long chain
  in milk sphingolipids 99–102
Biohydrogenation 13
Blood 9, 16–21
Breasts 3
Butyrate
  in milk triglycerides 62–63
  in rumen 12

Cancer, breast 2, 25, 27, 28, 66
Capillary endothelium 20
Cardiolipin 45, 64, 65, 85
Carotene 21, 74, 86
Casein 5, 6
Casein micelles 35, 36, 41
Casein synthesis 35
Cell
  capillary endothelial 20
  mammary epithelial 22, 25, 29–34, 43, 46
Cells 2, 6, 11
  adipose 23–24
  de-differentiation 27
Ceramides 66
  milk 101
Cerebrosides 66
  milk 85, 99–101
Cholesterol 20, 31, 34, 49, 66–74, 94
  functions of 67
  in milk and milk products 77
  in various foods 77
  and sphingomyelin 68–69
  and structure of HDL 68

Cholesterol
  dietary 69
Cholesterol esters 68
  milk 73–74, 85, 102
Cholesterol metabolism 67–70
Cholesterol, milk 70–74, 85–86
  origin of 72–74
Cholesterol serum 69
Cholesterol synthesis 72
Chylomicrons 17
CoA esters 54, 56, 58
Colchicine 42, 47
Colostrum 7, 35
Crescents
  on fat globules 50
Cyclopropane acids 93
Cytosol 30

7-Dehydrocholesterol in milk 86
Dihydrolanosterol 85
Diglycerides (diacylglycerols), milk 83–84
DNA 2, 26
Dry milk 2

Endoplasmic reticulum 26, 27, 30, 44, 45
Energy metabolism 52, 53
Enzymes 11
  milk 75
Epithelium, mammary 22, 25, 29–34, 43, 46
Ergocryptine 20
Estrogen 26

Fat droplet formation 38–39
Fat globule membrane, milk 44, 45, 48–51
  composition of 98
  lipids in 86–87
Fat globule, milk 5
  compartmentation of 51–52
  formation of 36–39
  secretion of 42, 47
Fat, milk 36
  depressed 21
  odor from 63
  polyunsaturated 14–15
Fatty acid composition 7, 8
Fatty acid synthetase 38, 54

INDEX

Fatty acids 36
  analysis of 87–88
  branched, in milk lipids 89, 91
  C_{22}-C_{24} 66
  cyclohexyl, in milk lipids 93
  free in serum 21
  hydroxy, in milk lipids 92
  in milk cholesterol esters 102
  in milk phospholipids 95–100
  in milk sphingolipids 99–102
  monoenoic, in milk lipids 89
  odd carbon, in milk lipids 89
  of hay 13
  oxo- in milk 92
  patterns in milks 57–58
  rumen 13
  short chain 7, 8
  transport of 62
  unsaturated 7, 8, 13, 14
  unsaturated in milk lipids 89–91
  volatile 12
Fatty acids, milk 8, 19
  synthesis of 54–58
Flavor 2, 6, 15

Galactosyl transferase, UDP 36
Gangliosides 66
  milk 102
Gases
  blood 9
  rumen 12
Gland, mammary 22
Globulins 35, 36
Globulins, immune 6
Glucose 36
Glucose metabolism 53
Glucose-6-phosphatase 27
Glycerol 59, 61
Glycerol ethers, milk 84, 93, 96, 98
Glycerol kinase 60
Glycerol-3-phosphate 59, 65
Glycolipids
  synthesis of 66
Glycoproteins 46
Glycosyl transferase 66
Golgi apparatus 26, 28, 30, 31, 35, 36, 40–43, 44, 45
  secretory process of 46–47
Golgi vesicles 37

Heart disease 14
Hormones 26, 34
Hydrocarbons, milk 86
Hydrocortisone 26
β-hydroxybutyrate metabolism 56
Hydroxy fatty acids
  in milk sphingolipids 100

Immune globulins 6

Insulin 20, 26, 27
Intestinal mucosa 69
Ions 7

Kinase, protein 35

α-lactalbumin 5, 6, 35–36
β-lactoglobulin 5, 6
Lactones, aliphatic 57
Lactose 4, 5, 7, 41
Lactose synthesis 5, 36, 41
Lanosterol 85
Lecithin-cholesterol-acyl-transferase 68
Linoleate 7, 13, 14
Lipase 11
Lipase, lipoprotein 20, 22, 59, 60
Lipids, microbial 12–13
Lipids, milk
  composition of 77–103
  fatty acids in 77, 88–93, 103
  technological importance of 76
Lipogenesis in milk 75–76
Lipoprotein lipase 20, 22, 59, 60
Lipoproteins (see serum lipoproteins)
Liver, rat 27
London–Van der Waals forces 47
Lymph 25
Lysosomes 29, 30
Lysozyme 6

Malonyl CoA 54
Marine mammals 4, 7
Membrane(s) 26, 27, 29–34, 36
  aging of 31–32
  composition of 43–46
  Golgi 44, 45, 66
  hepatocyte 68–69
  in milk 75
  in skim milk 42, 44
  lipids in 44, 45
  milk fat globule 48–51, 86–87
  origin of 75
  plasma 25, 30, 32
  preparation of 43
  protein in 46
  red blood cell 49
  sidedness of 50–51, 66
  transformation and flow of 31–32, 40
  vectoring of products in 30–32
Metabolism, general 8–11
Methyl ketones 57
Micelles, casein 6
Microtubules 42, 47
Microvilli 24
  in milk 42, 77
Milk
  components of 4
  nature of 3
  nutritive value of lipids in 76–77
  species variations 3, 4, 7

INDEX

Mitochondria 30, 56
Mitochondria, mammary 45
Monoglycerides 20, 21

5′Nucleotidase 49, 50–51
Nucleotide pyrophosphatase 50
Nucleus 30

Orotic acid 18, 77
Oxygenated fatty acids 57
Oxytocin 9, 24

Phenylacetic acid 16
3-Phenylpropionic acid 16
Phosphatidic acid 60, 65
Phosphatidylcholine 64, 65, 84, 95–98
　in triglyceride synthesis 62
Phosphatidylethanolamine 52, 65, 84, 95–98
Phosphatidylglycerol 64, 65
Phosphatidylinositol 65, 84, 95
Phosphatidylserine 52, 65, 84, 95
Phospholipids 32–34, 44, 45
　milk 21, 70, 71, 76, 84, 85, 95
　synthesis of 63–64
Phospholipids, milk
　composition of 84–85, 95–102
　fatty acids in 95–98, 100–102
Phosphopeptides 35
Phytanic acid 15, 91, 95
Plasma membrane 44, 45, 47, 48–51, 62, 64, 66
　sidedness of 50–52
Plasmalogens, milk 96, 98
Polyunsaturated milk fat 14–15, 93–94
Potassium 7
Progesterone 26
Prolactin 20, 26, 27, 28, 34
Propionate 12
Prostaglandin 26
Protected milk fat 14–15, 259–260
Proteins, milk 6–7, 35
Protozoa, rumen 11, 13

Refsums disease 16
Ribosomes 30
RNA 26, 30, 34, 35
Rumen 11–16

Salts, milk 7
Secretion of milk 39–42
Serum albumin 7, 18
Serum cholesterol 77
Serum free fatty acids 21

Serum lipoproteins 16–21
　and milk cholesterol 73
　composition 17, 19
　high density (HDL) 17–20, 68, 73
　low density (LDL) 17–20, 73
　very low density (VLDL) 17–20, 37, 69, 73
Serum triglycerides 19
Sex 3
Sialicic acid 44, 66
β-Sitosterol 85
Skim milk, membranes in 42, 44, 48–50
Sodium ions 7
Spermidine 27, 35
Sphingolipids, milk 84–85
　composition of 99–102
　fatty acids in 99–102
Sphingomyelin 32–34, 44, 45, 51, 64, 65, 66, 84, 85, 95, 99–102
Sphingosines 64, 65
　in milk sphingolipids 99, 101–102
Squalene 72, 86
Stearic acid 13
Stearyl desaturase 37, 55
Sterol esters, milk 102
Sterols, milk 85–86

Transferase, UDP-Galactosyl 36
Triglycerides, 36–39
　analysis of 79–82
　in blood 19, 60–61
Triglyceride synthesis 58
　glycerol-3-phosphate pathway 59, 65
　hydroxy acetone phosphate pathway 62
　in milk 75
　monoglyceride pathway 60–62
Triglycerides (triacylglycerols), milk 19, 21, 78–83
　acyl carbons in 63
　butyrate in 62–63
　position of fatty acids in 82
　structure of 81–83, 97
Triglycerides, serum 19

Vaccenic acid 13
Vincristine 42
Viruses 2
Vitamin A (Retinol) 74–75
　and secretion 75

Whey proteins 6